URTICARIA

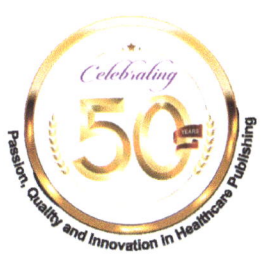

URTICARIA

Second Edition

Editor
Kiran V Godse MD PhD FRCP (Glasgow)
Professor
Department of Dermatology
DY Patil Hospital
Navi Mumbai, Maharashtra, India

Foreword
Hemangi Jerajani

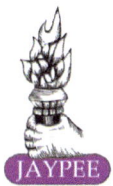

JAYPEE BROTHERS MEDICAL PUBLISHERS
The Health Sciences Publisher
New Delhi | London | Panama

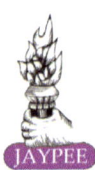 **Jaypee Brothers Medical Publishers (P) Ltd**

Headquarters
Jaypee Brothers Medical Publishers (P) Ltd
4838/24, Ansari Road, Daryaganj
New Delhi 110 002, India
Phone: +91-11-43574357
Fax: +91-11-43574314
Email: jaypee@jaypeebrothers.com

Overseas Offices
J.P. Medical Ltd
83 Victoria Street, London
SW1H 0HW (UK)
Phone: +44 20 3170 8910
Fax: +44 (0)20 3008 6180
Email: info@jpmedpub.com

Jaypee-Highlights Medical Publishers Inc
City of Knowledge, Bld. 235, 2nd Floor
Clayton, Panama City, Panama
Phone: +1 507-301-0496
Fax: +1 507-301-0499
Email: cservice@jphmedical.com

Jaypee Brothers Medical Publishers (P) Ltd
Bhotahity, Kathmandu, Nepal
Phone: +977-9741283608
Email: kathmandu@jaypeebrothers.com

Website: www.jaypeebrothers.com
Website: www.jaypeedigital.com

© 2019, Jaypee Brothers Medical Publishers

The views and opinions expressed in this book are solely those of the original contributor(s)/author(s) and do not necessarily represent those of editor(s) of the book.

All rights reserved. No part of this publication may be reproduced, stored or transmitted in any form or by any means, electronic, mechanical, photocopying, recording or otherwise, without the prior permission in writing of the publishers.

All brand names and product names used in this book are trade names, service marks, trademarks or registered trademarks of their respective owners. The publisher is not associated with any product or vendor mentioned in this book.

Medical knowledge and practice change constantly. This book is designed to provide accurate, authoritative information about the subject matter in question. However, readers are advised to check the most current information available on procedures included and check information from the manufacturer of each product to be administered, to verify the recommended dose, formula, method and duration of administration, adverse effects and contraindications. It is the responsibility of the practitioner to take all appropriate safety precautions. Neither the publisher nor the author(s)/editor(s) assume any liability for any injury and/or damage to persons or property arising from or related to use of material in this book.

This book is sold on the understanding that the publisher is not engaged in providing professional medical services. If such advice or services are required, the services of a competent medical professional should be sought.

Every effort has been made where necessary to contact holders of copyright to obtain permission to reproduce copyright material. If any have been inadvertently overlooked, the publisher will be pleased to make the necessary arrangements at the first opportunity. The **CD/DVD-ROM** (if any) provided in the sealed envelope with this book is complimentary and free of cost. **Not meant for sale.**

Inquiries for bulk sales may be solicited at: jaypee@jaypeebrothers.com

Urticaria

First Edition: 2016
Second Edition: **2019**

ISBN 978-93-5270-611-2

Contributors

Ana M Giménez-Arnau
Professor
Department of Dermatology
Hospital del Mar, IMIM
Universitat Autònoma
Barcelona, Spain

Andaç Salman
Department of Dermatology
Marmara University School of Medicine
Istanbul, Turkey

Clive EH Grattan
Consultant Dermatologist
St John's Institute of Dermatology
London, UK

Frank Siebenhaar
Department of Dermatology and Allergy
Charite Universitatsmedizin Berlin
Chariteplatz 1
Berlin, Germany

Isabel Ogueta C
Department of Dermatology
Hospital del Mar, IMIM
Universitat Autònoma
Barcelona, Spain

Department of Dermatology
Faculty of Medicine
Pontificia Universidad Católica de Chile
Región Metropolitana, Chile

Kiran V Godse
Professor
Department of Dermatology
DY Patil Hospital
Navi Mumbai, Maharashtra, India

Marcus Maurer
Professor
Department of Dermatology and Allergy
Charite Universitatsmedizin Berlin
Chariteplatz 1
Berlin, Germany

Martin K Church
Professor
Department of Dermatology and Allergy
Charite Universitatsmedizin Berlin
Chariteplatz 1
Berlin, Germany

Torsten Zuberbier
Professor
Department of Dermatology and Allergy
Charite Universitatsmedizin Berlin
Chariteplatz 1
Berlin, Germany

Foreword

I have a great pleasure in writing the foreword for the book on *Urticaria* edited by Dr Kiran V Godse. It is the second edition meant for the Dermatologists and Allergy Specialists.

Urticaria is a very common symptom and most people encounter this problem in their life, some having more symptoms than other. The treatment of urticaria has evolved over many years and each year—newer and effective drugs are indicated for its management. Autoimmunity plays a major role in causation of urticaria. Advent of biologics has changed the dynamics of treatment strategies of urticaria.

He has single-mindedly focused on urticaria since 2010 when he was made the SIG Urticaria Coordinator when I was the President of Indian Association of Dermatologists, Venereologists and Leprologists (IADVL). His team had prepared educational pamphlets and Consensus Statements for Indian Dermatologists.

He is a member of EAACI/GA^{2}LEN/EDF/WAO guidelines, which are endorsed in more than 40 societies of the World.

He has an excellent team of international and eminent writers on his team. He has compiled a classic book on urticaria with modern outlook. I wish him success in this endeavor.

Hemangi Jerajani
Professor and Head
Department of Dermatology
Mahatma Gandhi Memorial Medical College and Hospital
Navi Mumbai, Maharashtra, India
Director
International League of Dermatological Societies (ILDS)
(South-East Asia, Middle East and Africa)
Past President
IADVL (2010–11)

Preface to the Second Edition

It gives me immense pleasure to present this book of urticaria. The idea of writing this book was given to me by friends and colleagues. The book is concise book for ready reference. Six international authors have written seven chapters in this book. Our understanding of urticaria has changed in last two decades. Biologics have changed the treatment algorithm.

The book will be useful for busy practicing dermatologists, residents, and allergy specialists.

I wish to thank Sanofi Pharma for supporting this venture.

I wish to thank my family—Drs Meenal, Gauri, and Atharva for supporting me.

I wish to thank DY Patil Hospital staff for constant encouragement.

Kiran V Godse

Preface to the First Edition

It gives me great pleasure to present this book *Urticaria*. The Special Interest Group (SIG) on Urticaria was formed in 2009 when Dr Hemangi Jerajani was the President of the Indian Association of Dermatologists, Venereologists and Leprologists (IADVL). In the last two years, SIG on Urticaria has published patient education pamphlets on this condition and also a consensus statement on the management of urticaria.

The idea of writing this book was given to me by my SIG colleagues and friends who opined that although there were many excellent monographs on this subject, very few books dealt with urticaria from the Indian perspective. In India, though there is no dearth of clinical material, expensive and extensive investigations are often not possible due to financial and logistic constraints.

Our understanding of urticaria has radically changed in the past two decades. For example, today, most cases of chronic urticaria are now accepted to have an autoimmune etiology, and immunomodulating drugs are increasingly being used in the treatment of this condition, frustrating to patient and clinician alike.

Biologics, also known as biologic therapies or biological response modifiers, are drugs derived from living material (human, animal, or microorganism) like omalizumab. These have now been approved for treatment of chronic urticaria.

This book is meant to be companion of busy practicing dermatologists, residents and family physicians.

We are fortunate to have renowned international contributors who have authored four chapters in this book.

We have added four new chapters to this edition of book.

I would appreciate feedback from readers about the contents and presentation so that improvement can be made in future editions.

I wish to thank UCB Pharma for wholeheartedly supporting this venture. Finally, I wish to thank my wife Dr Meenal and children Gauri and Atharva for supporting my academic pursuits at the cost of family life.

I would be remiss if I did not acknowledge my teachers Dr Leslie Marquis, Dr Satish Wadhwa, Dr Srilata Trasi, and Dr Uday Khopkar who have made me what I am today in dermatology. Their debt cannot be lightly forgotten.

Last but not least, I wish to thank Dr Vijay Patil, President of DY Patil Group and Dean and staff of DY Patil Hospital for constant encouragement for my academic pursuits.

Kiran V Godse

Contents

1. **Classification of Urticaria** — 1
   Torsten Zuberbier

2. **Diagnosis of Urticaria** — 5
   Marcus Maurer

3. **Contact Urticaria: An Update** — 20
   Isabel Ogueta C, Ana M Giménez-Arnau

4. **Chronic Inducible Urticaria** — 28
   Andaç Salman, Ana M Giménez-Arnau

5. **Angioedema** — 44
   Clive EH Grattan

6. **Cutaneous Mastocytosis** — 54
   Frank Siebenhaar

7. **Pharmacology of Antihistamines** — 62
   Martin K Church

8. **Treatment of Chronic Spontaneous Urticaria** — 69
   Kiran V Godse

Annexure — 77

Index — 79

CHAPTER 1

Classification of Urticaria

Torsten Zuberbier

INTRODUCTION

This chapter is based on the latest EAACI/GA²LEN/EDF/WAO guidelines (2017) which classify urticaria based on clinical symptoms, duration, and frequency. Because of the overlap between the underlying mechanisms of the different subtypes of urticaria, a classification based on the underlying mechanisms—which was attempted earlier—is less useful.

Urticaria has been described as a medical entity since antiquity. However, only in the last century was there a better understanding of the different subtypes showing the high heterogeneity the disease. Misnomers such as urticaria pigmentosa, which in fact is a cutaneous manifestation of mastocytosis revealed. Similar to urticaria vasculitis, these diseases due to historical reasons are still often addressed in urticaria book chapters but in this case the wheal-like symptoms are not true wheals since they last longer and are not histamine-mediated but based on the true vasculitis occurring in superficial cutaneous vessels.

Furthermore, it needs to be noted that the symptom of urticaria—the wheal—can also occur under other circumstances as kind of bystander effect, such as in acute anaphylaxis or in association with syndromes such as Muckle-Wells syndrome.

Thus, in conclusion, an important aspect in the guideline work was first of all to have clear-cut definitions of the disease and its symptoms, always remembering that overlap is possible in the classical medical nomenclature. This also holds true for the term angioedema, which can be histamine-induced associated with urticaria or even the sole manifestation of urticaria, but can also occur due to bradykinin formation, e.g. in hereditary angioedema or in other, unrelated dermatological diseases as a symptom, such as in cheilitis granulomatosa.

Urticaria is a disease characterized by the appearance of wheals, angioedema or both, encompassing several subtypes. Diagnosis and treatment vary according to the subtype, so classification is important. The symptoms of urticaria (wheals and/or angioedema) can also occur in other conditions or diseases, e.g. anaphylaxis.

Wheals are itchy or burning swellings, variable in size, often surrounded by reflex erythema and of a fleeting nature, lasting anywhere from 1 to 24 hours before disappearing.

Angioedema is defined as sudden, pronounced swelling of the lower dermis and subcutis, sometimes painful rather than itchy and taking up to 72 hours to resolve. Angioedema frequently involves the mucous membranes (Flowchart 1.1).

Urticaria

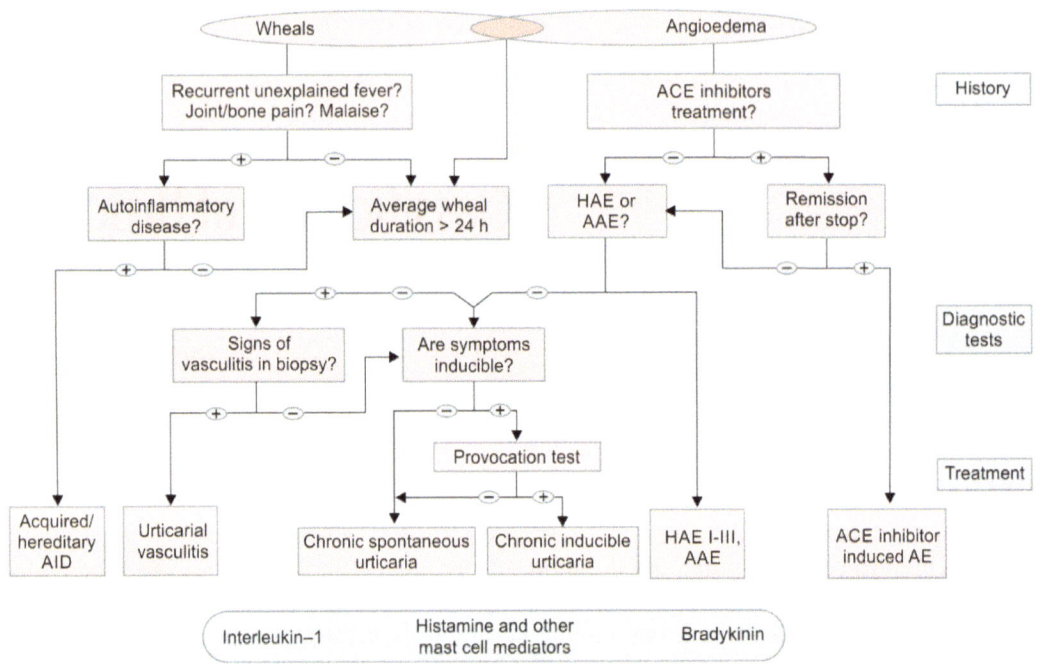

Flowchart 1.1: Differential diagnosis.

(AID: autoinflammatory disease; AE: angioedema; AAE: acquired angioedema; ACE: angiotensin-converting enzyme; HAE: hereditary angioedema)
Source: Zuberbier T, Aberer W, Asero R, et al. The EAACI/GA²LEN/EDF/WAO guideline for the definition, classification, diagnosis and management of urticaria. Allergy. 2018;73(7):1393-414.

CLASSIFICATION OF URTICARIA

Old systems of classification in urticaria were often driven by pathophysiology, e.g. classifying urticaria in allergic urticaria, urticaria due to infectious agents, or autoimmune urticaria. With a better understanding of the pathophysiology, this is no longer useful, since there is a high overlap between the different forms in the underlying pathophysiology. For example, allergic urticaria can occur in acute and chronic urticaria forms, and contact urticaria just to name some, and the same holds true for the term "autoimmune urticaria," which was originally devised when high-affinity IgE-receptor antibodies were discovered in chronic urticaria (Hide et al.). With the progress and knowledge it now becomes apparent that also other subtypes, e.g. cholinergic urticaria, autoimmune phenomena appear to be playing a role. Based on these considerations, the current guidelines classified urticaria based on the clinical manifestation, which makes it much easier for the practicing doctor to better diagnose the patients. In this classification, of course, there are also sometimes points that need to be discussed for better understanding. Thus, the term chronic urticaria is strictly reserved for the spontaneous appearance of wheals (to better show this, the term chronic spontaneous urticaria was introduced) but this does not mean that the physical subtypes of urticaria are not chronic; in these cases, symptoms are not chronic but only visible when physical stimuli are present.

Table 1.1 summarizes the classification. Note that the clinical manifestations of urticaria are broad and patients may exhibit two or more subtypes at one time.

Table 1.1: Symptomatic dermographism.

Chronic urticaria subtypes

Chronic spontaneous urticaria (CSU)	Inducible urticaria
Spontaneous appearance of wheals, angioedema or both for >6 weeks due to known[a] or unknown causes	Symptomatic dermographism[b] Cold urticaria[c] Delayed pressure urticaria[d] Solar urticaria Heat urticaria[e] Vibratory angioedema Cholinergic urticaria Contact urticaria Aquagenic urticaria

[a] For example, autoreactivity, that is the presence of mast cell-activating autoantibodies.
[b] Also called *urticaria factitia* or dermographic urticaria.
[c] Also called cold contact urticaria.
[d] Also called pressure urticaria.
[e] Also called heat contact urticaria.

Box 1.1: Diseases related to urticaria for historical reasons and syndromes including urticaria and/or angioedema.

- Maculopapular cutaneous mastocytosis (urticaria pigmentosa)
- Urticarial vasculitis
- Bradykinin-mediated angioedema (e.g. HAE)
- Exercise-induced anaphylaxis
- Cryopyrin-associated periodic syndromes (CAPS: urticarial rash, recurrent fever attacks, arthralgia, eye inflammation, fatigue and headaches), that is familial cold autoinflammatory syndrome (FCAS), Muckle-Wells syndrome (MWS) or neonatal-onset multisystem inflammatory disease (NOMID).
- Schnitzler's syndrome (recurrent urticarial rash and monoclonal gammopathy, recurrent fever attacks, bone and muscle pain, arthralgia or arthritis and lymphadenopathy)
- Gleich's syndrome (episodic angioedema with eosinophilia)
- Well's syndrome (granulomatous dermatitis with eosinophilia/eosinophilic cellulitis)
- Bullous pemphigoid (prebullous stage)

Some conditions formerly classified as urticaria are no longer considered to be subtypes of urticaria. These include "urticaria pigmentosa" (cutaneous mastocytosis), urticarial vasculitis, familial cold urticaria, and non-histaminergic angioedema (hereditary or acquired angioedema). Some subtypes of urticaria appear in conjunction with other syndromes such as Muckle-Wells (Box 1.1).

In order to properly classify urticaria, the following factors must be taken into consideration (*see* Flowchart 1.1 on differential diagnosis).

- Are there physical triggers or other external factors? If so, measure the intensity of the eliciting factor, e.g. how long does pressure need to be applied, and how much, in pressure urticaria; or temperature and time of exposure in cold urticaria.
- For nonphysical urticarias, guidelines suggest a unified scoring system from 0 (no wheals) to 3 (intense, many wheals, longer than 24 hours).
- Ask patients to record their symptoms and self-evaluate according to the scoring system. Self-evaluation is important since intensity fluctuates over the course of 24 hours. The self-evaluation can be supported by a periodic or one-time medical examination to ensure objectivity in the self-scoring.

GENERAL ISSUES

Wheal size sometimes indicates the severity of the disease; larger wheals means the urticaria is more severe and harder to treat. Wheal color may also help in diagnosis, as lighter colored wheals with a pink erythema indicate the involvement of histamine; the pink erythema is the result of dilatation of cutaneous vessels. Dark red or violaceous wheals are associated with vascular damage and leakage, perhaps indicating urticaria vasculitis.

Last but not least, it is also important to monitor disease intensity and appearance of wheals during the course of treatment (Mlynek, Weller). Very often, comparison pre- and post-treatment may also reveal factors indicating the underlying course. Ideally, this evaluation should be accompanied by the evaluation of the quality of life for which specialized instruments have been devised for urticaria (Baiardini).

BIBLIOGRAPHY

1. Baiardini I, Giardini A, Pasquali M, et al. Quality of life and patients' satisfaction in chronic urticaria and respiratory allergy. Allergy. 2003;58(7):621-3.
2. Hide M, Francis DM, Grattan CE, et al. Autoantibodies against the high-affinity IgE receptor as a cause of histamine release in chronic urticaria. N Engl J Med. 1993;328(22):1599-604.
3. Mlynek A, Zalewska-Janowska A, Martus P, et al. How to assess disease activity in patients with chronic urticaria? Allergy. 2008;63(6):777-80.
4. Weller K, Groffik A, Church MK, et al. Development and validation of the Urticaria Control Test: a patient-reported outcome instrument for assessing urticaria control. J Allergy Clin Immunol. 2014;133(5):1365-72.
5. Zuberbier T, Aberer W, Asero R, et al. The EAACI/GA^{2}LEN/EDF/WAO Guideline for the definition, classification, diagnosis and management of urticaria. Allergy. 2018;73(7):1393-414.
6. Zuberbier T, Aberer W, Asero R, et al. The EAACI/GA(2) LEN/EDF/WAO Guideline for the definition, classification, diagnosis, and management of urticaria: the 2013 revision and update. Allergy. 2014;69(7):868-87.

CHAPTER 2

Diagnosis of Urticaria

Marcus Maurer

INTRODUCTION

Urticaria is a heterogeneous group of diseases with several subtypes. Almost all types of urticaria present with a common and distinctive clinical pattern, i.e. itchy wheals and/or angioedema, with the exception of symptomatic dermographism (in which angioedema is absent) and pressure urticaria (in which there are no wheals). Diagnosing urticaria largely relies on the clinical picture and patient history. Diagnostic procedures are aimed at the identification of possible trigger factors and allergies in acute urticaria, at finding comorbidities and conditions that are relevant for the pathogenesis in chronic spontaneous urticaria (CSU) (as this can change therapeutic strategies and allow for a targeted treatment in some patients) and at characterizing the factors that induce physical urticarias (as avoiding them can lead to significant improvement or even total prevention of symptoms).

ACUTE SPONTANEOUS URTICARIA

Unless allergic urticaria is suspected, there is no need for a diagnostic work-up in patients with acute spontaneous urticaria (ASU). The diagnosis of ASU is primarily based on a thorough history, which should cover possible trigger factors,[1] such as infections (e.g. acute viral upper respiratory infections), medications (e.g. nonsteroidal analgesic drugs), and foods. According to the current EAACI/GA^{2}LEN/EDF/WAO guidelines on urticaria, further diagnostic tests are not generally recommended, due to the short disease duration—6 weeks maximum—and the self-limited course. Only a history pointing to relevant sensitizations to type I allergens, e.g. to foods or drugs, should prompt skin prick testing and measurements of specific immunoglobulin E (IgE). Even though viral infections are a frequent cause of ASU, taking blood samples for the determination of antiviral antibodies is not recommended due to low specificity.

CHRONIC SPONTANEOUS URTICARIA

Diagnostic procedures in CSU are performed to identify conditions that contribute to the pathogenesis of the disease as well as comorbidities, as treating them can help to reduce the burden of CSU. CSU, in most patients is an autoimmune disorder, with IgE autoantibodies to autoallergens (type I) or IgG autoantibodies that activate skin mast cells (type IIb).[2] Diagnostic measures to identify autoimmune type I or type IIb CSU patients are limited. As of now, it is not possible to measure IgE autoantibodies against self or autoantibodies directed against the high affinity IgE receptor (FcεRI) or against IgE itself in routine clinical practice.

The autologous serum skin test (ASST) is a screening test for type IIb autoimmune CSU. Detailed recommendations on how to perform and assess the ASST have been published.[3] Briefly, serum is acquired by centrifugation of freshly obtained whole blood. 50 μL of this serum is injected (intracutaneously) into the volar skin of the forearm. Testing of histamine and saline solution as positive and negative controls, respectively, should be done at the same time as serum testing and the responses should be read after 15 minutes (Fig. 2.1). A minimum difference of 1.5 mm in mean perpendicular wheal diameter between the autologous serum-induced response and the saline-induced response defines a positive response.[3] Where and when available, in vitro basophil histamine release assays or activation tests are useful for screening CSU patients for type IIb autoimmune CSU.[4,5]

In addition, one or both of the following common conditions are relevant in many patients: (i) infection and (ii) intolerance to food components or drugs.[1,6] Patients suffering from CSU are highly affected by the disease[7] and disease activity, disease control and the impairment of quality of life should be assessed routinely. Direct and indirect healthcare costs are significant, as the disease leads to 20–30% diminished job performance by patients.[8]

A search for relevant conditions, comorbidities and triggers should be conducted especially in patients who present with relapsing symptoms for more than 1 year and/or with high disease activity. CSU disease activity can be evaluated using the "urticaria activity score" (UAS), which is a clinical symptom score that combines daily recordings of the numbers of wheals and the intensity of pruritus[9] (for more details see further).

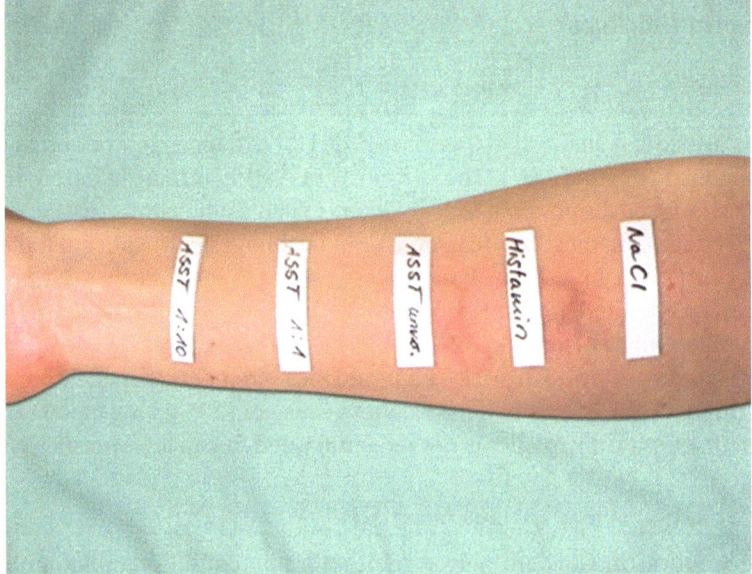

Fig. 2.1: Positive autologous serum skin test (ASST) in a patient with autoreactive chronic spontaneous urticaria: A big wheal developed where the patient's undiluted serum was injected 5 minutes earlier.

Diagnosis of Urticaria

Box 2.1: Items of interest in the clinical history of patients with chronic spontaneous urticaria (CSU).[6,7]

- First onset of CSU (Life events?)
- Frequency, duration, severity, shape, size, and localization of wheals
- Relevance of symptoms with time of day, day of week (weekend?), season (vacation?), menstrual cycle
- Presence of angioedema, subjective symptoms of lesion (itch, pain) or systemic manifestations (headache, gastrointestinal symptoms, joint pain, etc.)
- Family history of urticaria or/and atopy
- Previous or current allergies, intolerances, infections, and systemic illnesses
- Psychosomatic and psychiatric diseases
- Surgical implantation and events during surgery
- Gastric or intestinal problems (stool, flatulence)
- Possible precipitating factors (physical stimuli, exercise, stress, food, and medications).
- Use of medications (NSAIDs, injections, immunizations, hormones, laxatives, suppositories, ear and eye drops, alternative remedies)
- Smoke, alcohol use, personal and social status, occupation, free-time activities
- Quality of life impairment, emotional impact
- Therapies that have been used, response to treatment.

(NSAIDs: nonsteroidal anti-inflammatory drugs)

Most importantly, a thorough medical history, including information on presumed triggering factors and important aspects of the course of the disease, should be obtained. The points that should be clarified are provided in Box 2.1.[10]

When indicated, skin provocation tests [e.g. cold, heat, ultraviolet (UV), pressure] as well as exercise tests should also be performed in order to verify or rule out inducible urticarias (note: antihistamines must be discontinued for at least 2–3 days).

Keeping a "urticaria diary" for several weeks can be very helpful: it should be used to document the frequency and intensity of disease symptoms (wheals, itch, swelling, systemic symptoms), possible relevance of food intake and other activities (e.g. physical or emotional stress), and the patient's medication.

When looking for relevant conditions, comorbidities and/or triggers (Box 2.2), the focus should be on intolerance to foods and bacterial infections.[6]

How to search for relevant food intolerance in patients with chronic spontaneous urticaria (CSU)?

In contrast to IgE-mediated allergies, food intolerance is a pseudoallergy: symptoms can be similar to those of immediate type I allergic reactions, but the pathomechanism does not involve IgE antibodies against food allergens. Thus, there are no laboratory markers or skin provocation tests available to prove that food intake triggers symptoms. The most frequent triggers in patients with CSU and food intolerance are aromatic substances such as flavoring agents, aromatic substances, preservatives, and artificial colors. However, it is often difficult for patients to know which food triggers are relevant, as symptoms may occur up to 12 hours after food intake.[6] Also, several food components may have to act together to trigger symptoms. Moreover, as pseudoallergic reactions are dose dependent, relevant food associated-triggers may be tolerated in low doses.

A 3-week pseudoallergen-free elimination diet can help to test CSU patients for food intolerance.[11,12] Patients need to be informed that the effects may not be seen until 10–14 days after the start of diet. Responses to the diet should be assessed by UAS measurements and by

> **Box 2.2:** Diagnostic procedures for CSU.[2,7]
>
> *Routine procedures:*
> - Objectification of urticarial symptoms (possibly with a photograph)
> - Urticaria calender, diary, patient questionnaires
>
> *Extended diagnostic procedures:*
> - Differential blood count, ESR, CRP
> - Omission of suspected drugs (e.g. NSAIDs)
> - Ruling out autoreactive CSU: Autologous serum skin test (ASST) (if positive, test serum for anti-IgE and anti-FcεRIα where indicated), thyroid hormones and autoantibodies (anti-TSH, anti-TPO, anti-Tg), antinuclear autoantibodies (ANA, MCAAs)
> - Ruling out infection-associated CSU: *Helicobacter pylori* test (stool, breath test), AST, hepatitis serology, stool for parasites and fungi, urine analysis, ENT, and dental examination
> - Ruling out CSU due to intolerance: Pseudoallergen- and histamine-low diet for 3–4 weeks, provocation with pseudoallergen- and histamine-rich food
> - Ruling out type I allergy: Skin prick test, total and specific IgE
> - Tryptase, as indication of severe systemic disease
> - Searching for chronic inflammatory conditions
> - If persistence of the same wheal for more than 24 hours: Lesional skin biopsy.
>
> (ANA: antinuclear antibodies; AST: antistreptolysin test; CRP: C-reactive protein; CSU: chronic spontaneous urticaria; ENT: ear-nose-throat; ESR: erythrocyte sedimentation rate; IgE: immunoglobulin E; MCAAs: mast cell-activating antibodies; NSAIDs: nonsteroidal anti-inflammatory drugs; Tg: thyroglobulin; TPO: thyroid peroxidase; TSH: thyroid-stimulating hormone).

comparing the use of on-demand antihistamine treatment during the week before and the last week of the diet. The UAS is based on the evaluation of numbers of wheals and the intensity of itching each using a 0–3 point scale. It is calculated as the daily sum of the wheal and itch score, with a maximum score of 6 points per day and 42 points per week (for the UAS7)[1] (Table 2.1).

A previously performed clinical trial showed that a pseudoallergen-free diet is a safe, healthy and low-cost method to identify patients with CSU and food intolerance.[13] During this diet, all food containing artificial colors, antioxidants, preservatives, flavoring agents, and histamine-rich foods are avoided (Table 2.2). The following terms on an ingredient list indicate the presence of food additives: E100-E1518, coloring, preservative, gelling agents, thickening agents, moisturizing agents, emulsifiers, flavor enhancer, antioxidants, separating agents, coating, artificial sweeteners, baking agents, stabilizers, flour treatment agents, modified starches, foaming agents, artificial aroma.[1] Antihistamines or corticosteroids should be taken only in case of high disease activity (e.g. UAS = 6) or in case of an emergency during the diet, in order not to interfere with its effects. If urticarial symptoms fail to improve, the physician should look carefully into possible mistakes made by the patient during the diet (ideally, patients are supervised and guided by a specialized dietician). If urticarial symptoms improve by 50% or more during the pseudoallergen-free diet, a provocation test may be performed in a hospital. This test consists of the intake of pseudoallergen-rich provocation meals under emergency standby and infusion therapy. Patients should be closely monitored for 24 hours after provocation (risk of delayed systemic reactions).[6,12,14]

How to search for relevant infections in patients with chronic spontaneous urticaria (CSU)?
Bacterial infections, as well as viral, fungal or parasitic infections can contribute to the pathogenesis of CSU. The current guideline-recommend tests, i.e. a differential blood count analysis as well as the determination of blood sedimentation rate and/or CRP, together

Table 2.1: Urticaria activity score (UAS).[1]

How many wheals have appeared during the last 24 hours?	Scoring
None	0
Mild (<20 wheals/24 hours)	1
Moderate (20–50 wheals/24 hours)	2
Intense (>50 wheals/24 hours)	3
How severe was the itching during the last 24 hours?	Scoring
None	0
Mild (present but not annoying or troublesome)	1
Moderate (troublesome but does not interfere with normal daily activity or sleep)	2
Intense (severe itch, which is sufficiently troublesome to interfere with normal daily activity or sleep)	3

Table 2.2: List of foods that should be avoided during a pseudoallergen-free diet in intolerance-related chronic spontaneous urticaria (CSU).[10]

Generally forbidden:
All food, which contains flavorings, preservatives, dyestuffs or antioxidants. Industrial processed food is under suspicion.

	Can be eaten	Avoid if possible
Basic food	Bread and buns without preservatives, sorghum, grit, potatoes, rice, durum noodles (without eggs), rice wafers (only rice and salt)	All other food (e.g. pasta products, egg noodles, cakes, pommes frites)
Fat	Butter, plant oils	All other fat (margarine, mayonnaise, etc.)
Milk products	Fresh milk, fresh cream (without carrageen), quark, natural yoghurt, fresh unseasoned cheese, few young gouda	All other milk products
Food of animal origin	Fresh meet, fresh unseasoned mincemeat, fresh self-made cold meat	All industrial processed food of animal origin, eggs, fish, shellfishes
Vegetable	All vegetable except the forbidden ones, salad (cleaned thoroughly), carrots, zucchini, Brussels sprouts, white cabbage, Chinese cabbage, broccoli, and asparagus	Artichokes, peas, mushrooms, pieplant, spinach, tomatoes, all processed tomatoes, olives, and paprika
Spices	Salt, sugar, chive, and onions	All other spices, garlic, herbs
Sweets	None	All sweets, including chewing gum and sweeteners
Beverages	Milk, mineral water, coffee, unflavored black tea	All other beverages, herbal tea, alcohol
Spreads	Honey and all previously mentioned (allowed) products	All other spreads

with a focused patient history can help to discover potentially relevant infections. When indicated, specific diagnostic measures such as testing for *Helicobacter pylori* (stool, breath test or demonstration of antigen/antibodies) should follow (extended diagnostic program).[11] Interdisciplinary cooperation with dentists and ear, nose and throat specialists and X-ray and serological analyze for streptococcal (antistreptolysin) or staphylococcal infection can help to identify bacterial infections of the nasopharynx, e.g. recurrent sinusitis or tonsillitis.[6,15,16] The spectrum and prevalence of infections in CSU patients, and thereby the diagnostic workup needed to detect them, is influenced by many factors including the age of patients and where they live. To arrive at the conclusion that an infection contributed to the pathogenesis in a CSU patient requires that symptoms disappear or significantly improve after successful treatment of the infection.[1,6,11]

INDUCIBLE URTICARIAS

Inducible urticaria is a heterogeneous group of urticarias, which includes physical urticarias, e.g. cold and heat contact urticaria, delayed pressure urticaria, symptomatic dermographism/urticaria factitia, solar urticaria, and vibratory urticaria/angioedema, as well as other inducible urticarias, such as cholinergic urticaria.

Cold Urticaria

A typical case of cold urticaria can easily be recognized by the patient history and can be confirmed by a simple cold stimulation test, during which an ice cube, melting in a see-through plastic bag, is placed on the skin for 5 minutes. 10 minutes after removal of the cube a local wheal will develop. Shorter or longer provocation times may be used for some patients, e.g. 30 seconds (in patients who are very sensitive or afraid of strong reactions) and up to 20 minutes (in patients with a positive history but no reaction after 5 minutes).

Other methods include testing with cool packs or cold water baths (e.g. an arm can be submerged in cold water at 5–10°C for 10 minutes) and TempTest® measurements (Fig. 2.2). Because of the risk of causing systemic reactions, cool packs, and cold water baths should be used with caution.

TempTest® is a Peltier effect-based cold provocation device that allows exposure of the skin to thermal elements with defined temperatures (Fig. 2.3).[17] It is, therefore, ideally suited for evaluating thresholds of both stimulation temperatures and times in cold urticaria patients[18] (Figs. 2.4A and B). TempTest® testing not only determines thresholds in untreated patients (usually between 16–25°C) but can also be used to monitor responses to treatment. Knowledge of temperature and exposure time thresholds can help patients to avoid risky situations in their daily lives.[19]

Patients with cold urticaria do not need extensive laboratory testing.[20,21] In patients with a history of cold-induced wheals and/or angioedema but negative cold stimulation tests, atypical cold urticaria and autoinflammatory conditions should be investigated by appropriate diagnostic measures.

Heat Contact Urticaria

The diagnostic method of choice, if heat contact urticaria is suspected, is skin testing with metal or glass cylinders filled with warm water or a warm water bath. TempTest® can also be used where available. Heat provocation testing is performed for 5 minutes with a temperature of 45° on the volar forearm. The provocation time and temperature can be adapted individually. If a palpable, clearly visible wheal and flare type skin reaction occurs, the test reaction is rated positive.

Diagnosis of Urticaria

Patient information	Instructions:
Name: Date of birth:	Perform testing as indicated and document presence (+) or absence (−) of wheal (W), erythema (E), pruritus (P) and/or angioedema (A) as well as date/time of testing and who performed the test.

1. Symptomatic dermographism (Urticaria factitia)
Testsite: Upper back / Volar forearm
Test: Moderate stroking of the skin with a blunt smooth object (e.g. closed ballpoint pen tip, wooden spatula) /dermographometer (36 g/mm²)
Reading time: 10 minutes after testing

W	P

Date/Time _____ Test done by _____
If wheal and pruritus: Test threshold with dermographometer →

2. Cold contact urticaria
Testsite: Volar forearm/abdomen
Test: Melting ice cube in thin plastic bag/TempTest (4°C) for 5 minutes
Reading times: 10 minutes after testing

W	P

Date/Time _____ Test done by _____
If wheal: Test cold stimulation time or temperature threshold →

3. Heat contact urticaria
Testsite: Volar forearm
Test: Heat source/TempTest (45°C) for 5 minutes
Reading times: 10 minutes after testing

W	P

Date/Time _____ Test done by _____
If wheal: Test cold stimulation time or temperature threshold →

4. Delayed pressure urticaria
Testsite: Shoulder/Upper Back/Thighs/Volar forearm
Test: Suspension of weights over shoulder (7 kg, shoulder strap width: 3 cm) for 15 minutes or weighted rods (1.5 cm diameter: 2.5 kg; or 6.5 cm diameter: 5 kg) for 15 min. Dermographometer at 100 g/mm² for 70 sec
Reading times: ≈6 hours after testing

A	E

Date/Time _____ Test done by _____
If angioedema: Test threshold →

5. Solar urticaria
Testsite: Buttocks
Test: UVA 6 J/cm² & UVB 60 mJ/cm² irradiation (e.g. Saalmann Multitester SBC LT 400) Visible light (projector)
Reading times: 10 minutes after testing

	W	P
UVA		
UVB		
Visible light		

Date/Time _____ Test done by _____
If wheal: Test threshold →

6. Vibratory urticaria/angioedema
Testsite: Volar forearm
Test: Vortex vibrator for 10 minutes, 1000 rpm
Reading times: 10 minutes after testing

A	P

Date/Time _____ Test done by _____

7. Cholinergic urticaria
Test 1: Exercise using a machine, e.g. bicycle trainer or treadmill, to the point of sweating, then continue for 15 minutes,

if positive test reaction:

Test 2: 42°C bath, monitor body temperature. Continue bath for 15 minutes after body temperature has increased by ≥ 1°C over baseline

Reading times: Immediately and 10 minutes after end of test

1. Exercise	W	P		2. Hot bath	W	P

If positive reaction →

Fig. 2.2: Provocation testing for physical and cholinergic urticarias.[19]

Threshold testings

1. Symptomatic dermographism (Urticaria factitia)

Testsite: Upper back
Test: Moderate stroking of the skin with a dermographometer
Reading times: 10 minutes after testing

g/mm²	20	36	60
P			
W			

Date/Time _____

Test done by _____

2. Cold contact urticaria

Testsite: Volar forearm
Test: TempTest®/water bath for 5 minutes, or melting ice cube
Reading times: 10 minutes after end of testing

Ice cube, stimulation time threshold testing

	30 sec	1 min	2 min	5 min
P				
W				

Date/Time _____

Test done by _____

TempTest®, temperature threshold testing

°C:	4	5	6	7	8	9	10	11	12	13	14	15	16	17	18	19
P																
W																

°C:	20	21	22	23	24	25	26	27	28	29	30	31	32	33	34	35
P																
W																

3. Heat contact urticaria

Testsite: Volar forearm
Test: Heat source/TempTest®, 5 minutes
Reading times: 10 minutes after testing

°C:	45	44	43	42	41	40	39	38	37	36
P										
W										

Date/Time _____

Test done by _____

4. Delayed pressure urticaria

Testsite: Volar forearm (rod), upper back (dermographometer)
Test: Weighted rods (6.5 cm diameter) for 15 minutes or Dermographometer at 100g/mm²
Reading times: ≈6 hours after testing

Weighted rod

kg:	1	2	3	4	5
A					
E					

Date/Time _____

Test done by _____

Dermographometer 100g/mm²

sec:	20	30	40	50	60
A					
E					

5. Solar urticaria

Testsite: Buttocks
Test: UVA & UVB irradiation (e. g. Saalmann Multitester SBC LT 400)
Reading times: 10 minutes after testing

UVA J/cm²	P	W
2,4		
3,3		
4,2		

Date/Time _____

Test done by _____

UVB mJ/cm²	P	W
24		
33		
42		

Fig. 2.3: Threshold testings for physical urticarias.[19]

Diagnosis of Urticaria

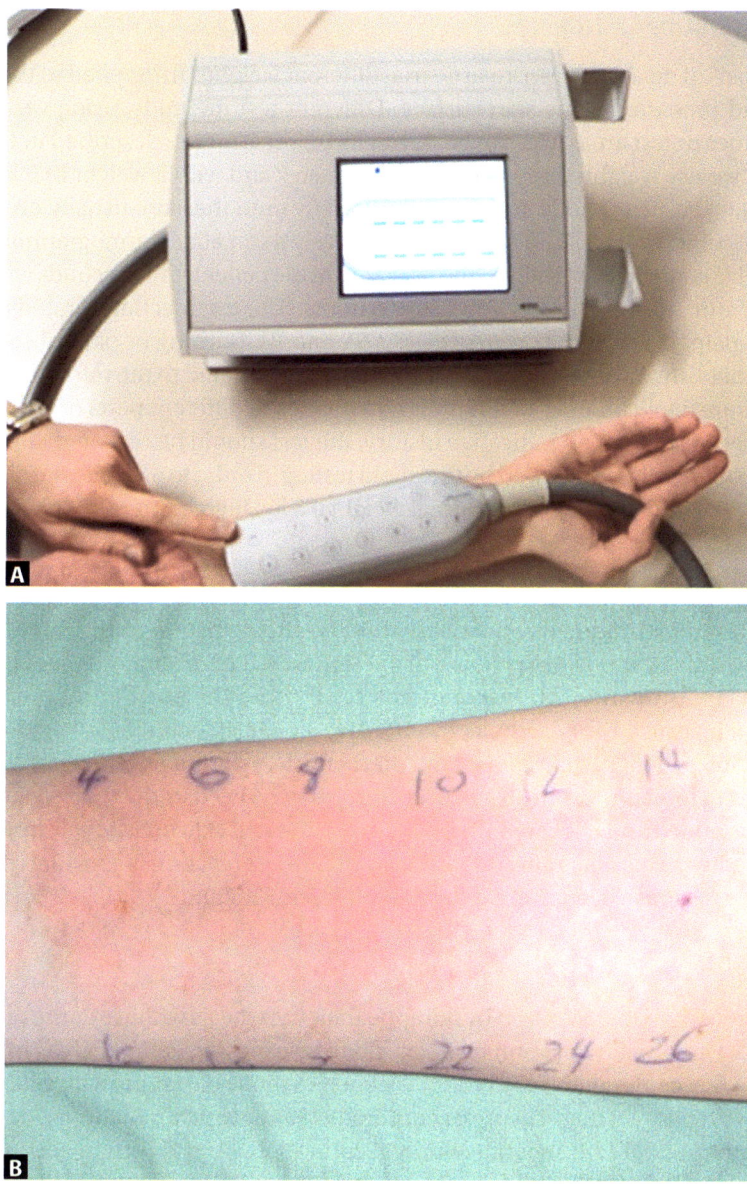

Figs. 2.4A and B: Use of the Temp*Test*® device to determine the threshold temperature in a patient with cold urticaria (A). The threshold temperature (i.e. the highest temperature tested that is sufficient to produce a wheal) in this patient is 14°C (B).

Additionally, a subjective evaluation of the intensity of itching should be done by the patient. After a positive heat provocation test, the threshold temperature should be determined. To this end, the occurrence of wheals and itching is determined 10 minutes after consecutive 5-minute provocations with temperatures between 45°C and 36°C. The determination of threshold temperature plays an important role for the evaluation of disease activity and the efficacy of initiated therapies.[11,18]

Delayed Pressure Urticaria

For the diagnosis of delayed pressure urticaria, different weights are applied to the skin, which exert a defined pressure on the skin surface. Different test methods, using various weights, application times or test areas, e.g. the back, thighs or forearms are described in the literature. In our center, we use weighted rods, 6.5 cm in diameter and with a weight of 5 kg, which is a pressure of 14.6 kPa. These rods are lowered vertically onto the skin, usually on the patient's forearm, for 15 minutes (Figs. 2.5A and B). Alternatively a so-called dermographometer can be used. This device is applied vertically to the back skin of the patient for 70 seconds with an applied force of 100 g/mm^2. Results are recorded after 6 hours. The test reaction is rated as positive, if a delayed red palpable swelling occurs (Figs. 2.5A and B). Burning or painful sensations can occur simultaneously. False negative test results might be related to the refractory period after previous pressure application or to different sensitivities in different parts of the body. In case of a negative test result, but an indicative history, the test should be repeated after 48 hours. A positive test result should be followed by threshold testing in order to evaluate the disease activity and the efficacy of initiated therapies (initial weight 0.5 kg, increments: 0.5 kg).[18,22]

Urticaria Factitia (Symptomatic Dermographism)

The most appropriate routine diagnostic method for the detection of urticaria factitia is the elicitation of wheals by moderate rubbing of the skin with a blunt smooth object, e.g. a closed ballpoint pen tip. Urticaria factitia symptoms result from the exertion of tangential shear forces on the skin, caused, for example, by intensive, linear scratching. Provocation should be performed on the patient's back or forearm. Alternatively, a dermographometer, which applies different forces to the skin—from 20 g to 60 g/mm^2, may be used. Individual trigger thresholds should be determined and it is very important, that the tested skin area is healthy and free from infections. Reading takes place after 10 minutes and the test reaction is considered positive, if a wheal and flare response occurs and if the patient reports itching[11,18,21] (Fig. 2.6).

Solar Urticaria

This form of urticaria is characterized by the appearance of wheals within minutes after exposure to sunlight[23,24] (Fig. 2.7). Provocation testing is done by exposing defined areas of the patient's skin (usually a few centimeters) to UV and visible radiation. UV lamps with filters (UV-A and UV-B) may be used for testing. The most common areas at which radiation is applied are the buttocks and they should be separately provoked in the UV-A (at 6 J/cm^2), UV-B (at 60 mJ/cm^2) and visible light range (e.g. slide projector at a 10 cm distance). In solar urticaria patients, a wheal and flare reaction appears at the test site 10 minutes after radiation. As in other forms of physical urticaria, threshold testing should be performed by varying the radiation dose or by changing the time of exposure to the light source (*see* Fig. 2.3). This will lead to information about disease activity and response to therapy.[18]

Cholinergic Urticaria and Exercise-induced Urticaria/Anaphylaxis

In cholinergic urticaria actively (e.g. due to exercise) or passively (e.g. having a hot bath) induced increases of the body temperature result in the appearance of itching and whealing (Fig. 2.8).

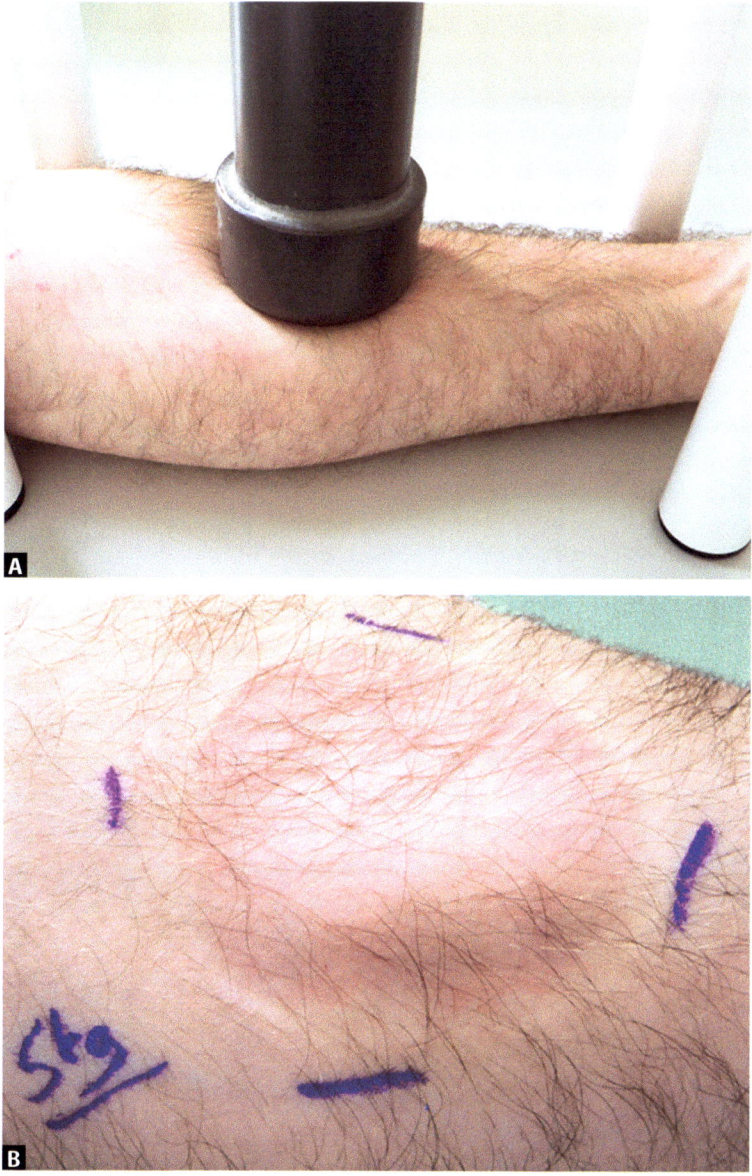

Figs. 2.5A and B: Pressure testing for delayed pressure urticaria (A). Swelling after application of 14.6 kPa pressure with a 5 kg heavy metal rod for 15 minutes (B).

Typically, the wheals are tiny, short-lived and accompanied by a pronounced flare reaction which is often localized on the limbs and trunk.[25,26] This form of urticaria should be differentiated from exercise-induced urticaria/anaphylaxis, in which exercise but not passive warming provokes symptoms (cutaneous and, more frequently than in cholinergic urticaria, systemic symptoms). In the differential diagnosis, attention should be given to food or drug-dependent exercise-induced anaphylaxis.[11]

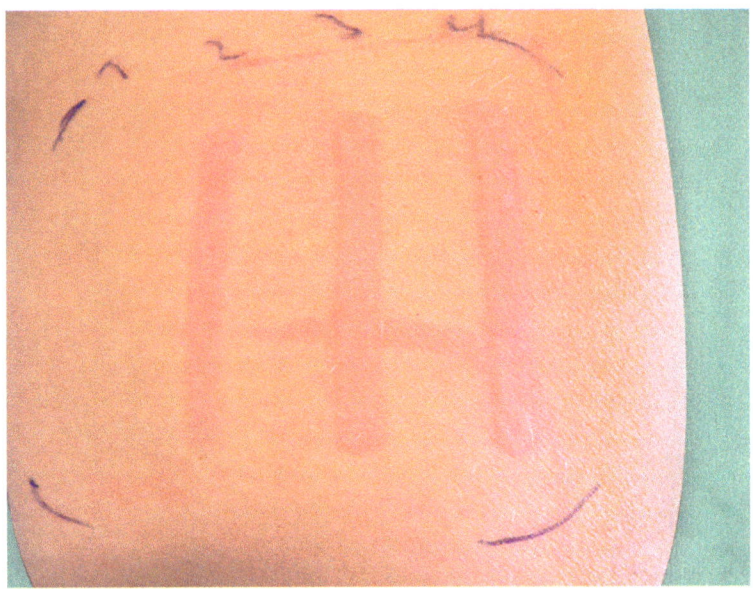

Fig. 2.6: A patient with urticaria factitia/symptomatic dermographism after testing with a dermographometer.

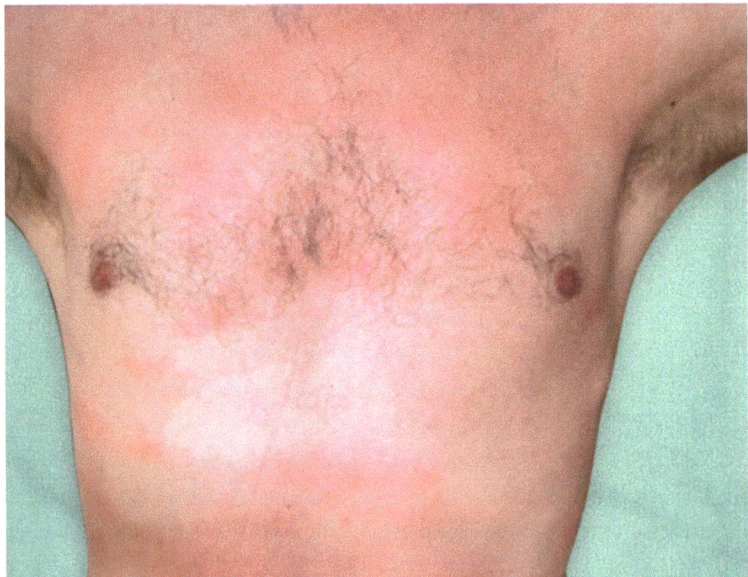

Fig. 2.7: A patient with solar urticaria, 15 minutes after provocation.

To differentiate cholinergic urticaria from exercise-induced urticaria a two-step approach should be carried out in terms of provocation testing. Moderate physical exercise, matching the patient's age and general condition, should be applied (e.g. on a stationary bicycle or on a treadmill). Patient should reach the point of sweating and continue for another 15 minutes. If this first step is positive, a passive warming test should be performed at least 24 hours later

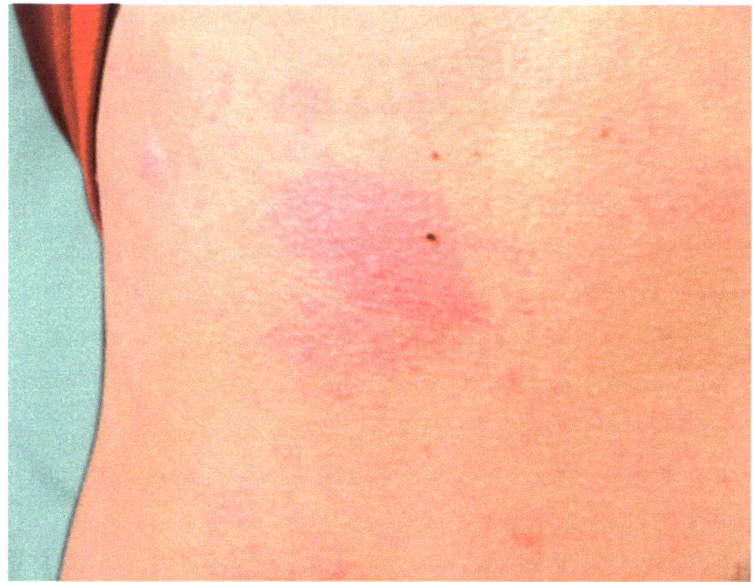

Fig. 2.8: A patient with cholinergic urticaria 15 minutes after bicycle riding.

(full bath at 42°C for up to 15 minutes until body core temperature rises more than 1°C), in order to rule out exercise-induced urticaria/anaphylaxis[18] (*see* Fig. 2.2). During provocation, a trained member of the team should always be present in case of an anaphylactic reaction. The patient's pulse, blood pressure, and peak flow rates should be monitored during provocation and emergency measures and equipment must be easily accessible.

Vibratory Urticaria/Angioedema

This rare type of physical urticaria is characterized by itching and swelling within minutes after local exposure to vibration.[27,28] A laboratory vortex mixer can be used as a provocation tool. The forearm is kept on a flat plate laid on the vortex mixer which is run between 780 rpm and 1380 rpm[29] for 10 minutes. After 10 minutes, the patient should be checked for swelling at the site of provocation.

AQUAGENIC URTICARIA

Aquagenic urticaria presents with urticarial symptoms after contact with water. Diagnostically, wet cloths at body temperature can be applied to the patient for 20 minutes.

CONTACT URTICARIA

Contact urticaria is an immediate but transient localized swelling/whealing response and redness that occurs on the skin after direct contact with an exogenous agent. If the eliciting factor is not clear from the patient's history, the following diagnostic steps should be taken: firstly, a patch test (open application or with occlusion) can be applied for 20 minutes on healthy and on previously damaged skin; the area should be examined after 30 minutes and after 24 hours if protein contact dermatitis is suspected. Secondly, a normal prick or patch test can be performed. Thirdly, the patient can be exposed in a controlled way, e.g. with latex gloves. Finally, specific IgE measurements can be helpful if doubts still remain.[30,31]

ACKNOWLEDGMENTS

This chapter is based in part on an earlier version co-authored by Nicole Schoepke, Georgios Doumoulakis, and Marcus Maurer.

REFERENCES

1. Zuberbier T, Grattan C, Maurer M. Urticaria and Angioedema. Berlin, Heidelberg: Springer-Verlag; 2010.
2. Maurer M, Metz M, Magerl M, et al. Autoreactive urticaria and autoimmune urticaria. Der Hautarzt. 2004;55:350-6.
3. Konstantinou GN, Asero R, Maurer M, et al. EAACI/GA(2)LEN task force consensus report: the autologous serum skin test in urticaria. Allergy. 2009;64:1256-68.
4. Deacock SJ. An approach to the patient with urticaria. Clin Exp Immunol. 2008;153:151-61.
5. Gimenez-Arnau A, Serra-Baldrich E, Camarasa JG. Chronic aquagenic urticaria. Acta Derm Venereol. 1992;72:389.
6. Maurer M, Grabbe J. Urticaria: its history-based diagnosis and etiologically oriented treatment. Dtsch Arztebl Int. 2008;105:458-65; quiz 465-6.
7. Maurer M, Ortonne JP, Zuberbier T. Chronic urticaria: an internet survey of health behaviours, symptom patterns and treatment needs in European adult patients. Br J Dermatol. 2009;160:633-41.
8. Delong LK, Culler SD, Saini SS, et al. Annual direct and indirect health care costs of chronic idiopathic urticaria: a cost analysis of 50 nonimmunosuppressed patients. Arch Dermatol. 2008;144:35-9.
9. Mlynek A, Zalewska-Janowska A, Martus P, et al. How to assess disease activity in patients with chronic urticaria? Allergy. 2008;63:777-80.
10. Zuberbier T, Chantraine-Hess S, Hartmann K, et al. Pseudoallergen-free diet in the treatment of chronic urticaria. A prospective study. Acta Derm Venereol. 1995;75:484-7.
11. Zuberbier T, Aberer W, Asero R, et al. The EAACI/GA²LEN/EDF/WAO guideline for the definition, classification, diagnosis and management of urticaria. The 2017 revision and update. Allergy. 2018;73:1393-414.
12. Maurer M, Hanau A, Metz M, et al. Relevance of food allergies and intolerance reactions as causes of urticaria. Der Hautarzt. 2003;54:138-43.
13. Magerl M, Pisarevskaja D, Scheufele R, et al. Effects of a pseudoallergen-free diet on chronic spontaneous urticaria: a prospective trial. Allergy. 2010;65:78-83.
14. Reese I, Zuberbier T, Bunselmeyer B, et al. Diagnostic approach for suspected pseudoallergic reaction to food ingredients. J Dtsch Dermatol Ges. 2009;7:70-7.
15. Hartmann K. Urticaria: Classification and diagnosis. Der Hautarzt. 2004;55:340-3.
16. Wedi B, Raap U, Wieczorek D, et al. Infections and chronic spontaneous urticaria. A review. Der Hautarzt. 2010;61:758-64.
17. Siebenhaar F, Staubach P, Metz M, et al. Peltier effect-based temperature challenge: An improved method for diagnosing cold urticaria. J Allergy Clin Immunol. 2004;114:1224-5.
18. Siebenhaar F, Weller K, Mlynek A, et al. Acquired cold urticaria: Clinical picture and update on diagnosis and treatment. Clin Exp Dermatol. 2007;32:241-5.
19. Magerl M, Altrichter S, Borzova E, et al. The definition, diagnostic testing and management of chronic inducible urticarias—The EAACI/GA²LEN/EDF/UNEV 2016 consensus panel recommendations 2016 update and revision. Allergy. 2016;71:780-802.

20. Kozel MM, Mekkes JR, Bossuyt PM, et al. The effectiveness of a history-based diagnostic approach in chronic urticaria and angioedema. Arch Dermatol. 1998;134:1575-80.
21. Kozel MM, Bossuyt PM, Mekkes JR, et al. Laboratory tests and identified diagnoses in patients with physical and chronic urticaria and angioedema: A systematic review. J Am Acad Dermatol. 2003;48:409-16.
22. Fleischer M, Grabbe J. Physical urticaria. Hautarzt. 2004;55:344-9.
23. Chong WS, Khoo SW. Solar urticaria in Singapore: an uncommon photodermatosis seen in a tertiary dermatology center over a 10-year period. Photodermatol Photoimmunol Photomed. 2004;20:101-4.
24. Guzelbey O, Ardelean E, Magerl M, et al. Successful treatment of solar urticaria with anti-immunoglobulin E therapy. Allergy. 2008;63:1563-5.
25. Czarnetzki BM. Ketotifen in cholinergic urticaria. J Allergy Clin Immunol. 1990;86:138-9.
26. Illig L. On the pathogenesis of cholinergic urticaria. I. Clinical observations and histological studies. Arch Klin Exp Dermatol. 1967;229:231-47.
27. Lawlor F, Black AK, Breathnach AS, et al. Vibratory angioedema: Lesion induction, clinical features, laboratory and ultrastructural findings and response to therapy. Br J Dermatol. 1989;120:93-9.
28. Mathelier-Fusade P, Vermeulen C, Leynadier F. Vibratory angioedema. Ann Dermatol Venereol. 2001;128:750-2.
29. Keahey TM, Indrisano J, Lavker RM, et al. Delayed vibratory angioedema: Insights into pathophysiologic mechanisms. J Allergy Clin Immunol. 1987;80:831-8.
30. Wakelin SH. Contact urticaria. Clin Exp Dermatol. 2001;26:132-6.
31. Gimenez-Arnau A, Maurer M, De La Cuadra J, et al. Immediate contact skin reactions, an update of contact urticaria, contact urticaria syndrome and protein contact dermatitis—"a never ending story". Eur J Dermatol. 2010;20:552-62.

CHAPTER 3

Contact Urticaria: An Update

Isabel Ogueta C, Ana M Giménez-Arnau

INTRODUCTION

Contact urticaria syndrome (CUS) is a syndrome characterized by an inflammatory skin response to diverse and specific agents that triggered different clinical types of immediate contact reactions (ICSR).[1] Systemic involvement can also be present, being manifested by asthma, conjunctivitis, rhinitis or other oropharyngeal symptoms, such as difficult swallowing, lip swelling and anaphylaxis.[2] Initially was described by Maibach and Johnson in 1975[3] and, since then, multiples environmental triggers have been described. We have learned that chemicals with low molecular weight and also proteins can induce ICSR in a range from immediate wheals immunoglobulin E (IgE)-mediated to immediate eczema, a lymphocyte driven cutaneous reaction.[4] So, in this way, the proteins (high molecular weight) and chemicals (low molecular weight) can induce ICSR, clinically expressed with wheals, pruritus and eczema, immediately after contact with the trigger, through an immunological or a nonimmunological mechanism still under study. These cutaneous lesions characterize two defined entities, contact urticaria (CoU), and protein contact dermatitis (PCD). Both can appear over normal or previously eczematous skin and, the trigger can induce both responses independently in the same patient.[5] Both diseases are included in the definition of CUS.[6]

Contact urticaria involves wheal and flare reaction following external contact with an environmental agent, appearing within 30 minutes and clearing completely within hours, without residual signs.[7] On the other hand, PCD was defined by Hjorth and Roed-Petersen in 1976 as an immediate dermatitis induced after contact with proteins. For example, they described cases in which patients suffering exacerbation of the itch at 10–30 minutes after contact with fish, meat, and vegetables, being followed by erythema and vesicles; when applied relevant food on affected skin, they saw urticaria or eczema. In these patients, an association with atopy close to 50% has been seen.[8-11]

The main goal of this chapter is to introduce the essentials and update concepts to understand a specific syndrome, which is often misdiagnosed.

DEFINITIONS

Immediate contact reactions is an inflammatory condition that appears within minutes of skin contact with multiples substances, such as proteins as food or vegetable or chemicals such as antibiotics, or cosmetics, for example. Clinically they are expressed as wheals, itch or eczema, characterizing two entities, CoU, and PCD, both with different physiopathological mechanisms, according with the trigger factor characteristics.[12] CUS involves both diseases, manifesting as wheals in CoU and eczema/dermatitis in the PCD cases, based on responsible trigger factor. So, the exposure to proteins or chemicals can induce wheals and also dermatitis or eczema. In any case, the clinical manifestation will be triggered after the immediate contact with the trigger and, sometimes, extracutaneous involvement is present.

The list of published products responsible for CoU or PCD is very long. Sometimes, the agent involved in the immediate reaction has been correctly studied and described: food and food additives, fragrances, animal and plant derivatives, cosmetics, preservatives, drugs, metals, occupational products, etc. The identification and knowledge of the responsible agent becomes mandatory based in the preventive treatment and also in the assessment of the occupational relevance.[13] Both CoU and especially PCD, characterized by chronic and recurrent dermatitis of the hands and forearm,[14] involve occupations where wet work, irritants substances exposure, food contact with cheese products, seafood products, flowers, veterinary products and glove occlusion is frequent.[15] In a 10-year retrospective study among 373 food handlers with occupational dermatoses in Denmark, show that 22% had PCD and only 2.4% CoU. In this patient group, prick by prick test was positive for fresh vegetables and greengrocers in the context of chronic hand eczema.[16] On the other hand, in the seafood industry has been reported occupational PCD in 3–11%.[17]

Historically, the lesions suggestive of contact dermatitis have been studied by patch test, as a manifestation of type IV hypersensitivity, nevertheless, for immediate contact dermatitis, such as CoU or PCD, which involves type I hypersensitivity IgE-mediated, the prick test is of choice for the study as a cutaneous provocation test.[18]

PHYSIOPATHOLOGY

The mechanisms underlying ICSR are different in CoU and PCD, being immunologic or nonimmunologic.

Nonimmunological CoU (NICoU) is more common because of *Urtica obonica* and it is characterize by vasogenic mediators, such as histamine, leukotrienes, acetylcholine, prostaglandins, etc. without involvement of immunological processes.[19] The endothelial damage is, i.e. caused by dimethyl sulfoxide (DMSO), inducing mast cell degranulation.[20] It has been seen a good therapeutic response in NICoU with nonsteroidal anti-inflammatory drugs[21] and acetylsalicylic acid,[22] suggesting a probable role for prostaglandins in the disease's pathogenesis. If topical benzoic peroxide or ascorbic acid is involved, there is prostaglandin D2 without histamine release the responsible.[23] For this reasons, antihistamines do not inhibit NICoU reactions. Symptoms are usually localized within contact area and depend on the nature of substance, concentration, vehicle, rout, and site of exposition. Generalized urticaria is very strange. For example, irritant products or proinflammatory mediator causing NICoU can be animal hair or spines plant. Other responsible agents of NICoU are preservatives, flavoring in cosmetics, topical medication, and fragrances; insecticides and laboratory chemicals also induce it, taking relevance in occupational dermatoses study, previously mentioned.

Immunological CoU (ICoU) is a type I hypersensitive reaction IgE-mediated, in which is necessary that patient is previously sensitized.[24] Sensitization can be through skin or respiratory/gastrointestinal mucosa. When exposed to specific allergen, IgE binding on mast cell and induces its degranulation, with release of histamine, leukotrienes, kinins, platelet-activated factor and prostaglandins. PCD is an eczematous IgE-mediated reaction through protein, as it happens in atopic dermatitis when aeroallergens exposure is the trigger. So, therefore, a combination of type I and IV hypersensitive reactions are suggested as PCD pathogenesis,[25] supported by positive prick test and also patch test.[26] Clinical manifestation can vary from localized hives, pruritus, erythema to, although rare, generalized urticaria, and anaphylactic shock.[27]

STAGES OF SEVERITY OF THE CONTACT URTICARIA SYNDROME

The CUS can be classified into different stages, according its severity.[28] When occurs only cutaneous reactions, the CUS is classified in stages 1 and 2.
- *Stage 1:* Involves eczema or immediate contact dermatitis, localized CoU, and symptoms such as pruritus or burning sensation.
- *Stage 2:* Refers to generalized urticaria after a local contact.
- *Stage 3 and 4:* Symptoms or extracutaneous reactions that can be part of a severe reaction. In the stage 3, can occur asthma, orolaryngeal symptoms or gastrointestinal illness; in stage 4, the reactions are more severe, such as anaphylactic or anaphylactoid reactions. On the other hand, CoU is potentially mortal; for example, the immediate contact with latex protein can produce anaphylaxis and even death.

DIAGNOSIS

The diagnosis of CUS is clinical. It includes signs and symptoms that define two entities, (1) CoU and (2) PCD, which showing different patterns of inflammation. Both diseases are characterized by ICSR: CoU shows immediate itchy hives and/or angioedema, which appear immediately after contact with suspect allergen, and PCD shows immediate itchy erythema, papules, vesicles, fissures, excoriation or lichenified skin. Both cases, the pruritus is the most important symptom. The CoU clinical aspect is similar from that of other type of urticaria, nevertheless, it can change according with the type of the contact trigger agent (lineal distribution if contact are plants, punctuate wheals if the allergen penetrate by follicles, etc.). In the PCD cases, within the term contact dermatitis, different types of skin lesions can be present, such as erosions, urticaria, eczema, lichenoid eruptions, erythroderma or photosensitive reactions.[29]

Wheals and/or angioedema are clinical lesions that define any type of urticaria. Wheals characterize by central swelling and surrounded erythema, burning sensation and fleeting nature.[30] The skin recovers its normal appearance within 1–24 hours, without residual lesions.[31] Angioedema is characterized by important erythema and subcutaneous edema. It resolves within 24–72 hours. Histologically, hives are characterized by edema in upper and mid-dermis, with venules and lymphatic vessels dilatation, without vessels wall necrosis. When angioedema occurs, primarily the lower dermis and subcutaneous are involved.[32] In the PCD cases, spongiosis of the epidermis is the defining pathologic of eczema, and the confluence of spongiosis lets see vesicles and bullae. When dermatitis is chronic, the skin becomes acanthotic.[33]

Contact urticaria and PCD belong to the first staging of the CUS. The same trigger agent (protein or low molecular weight substances) can induce both entities in the same patient,

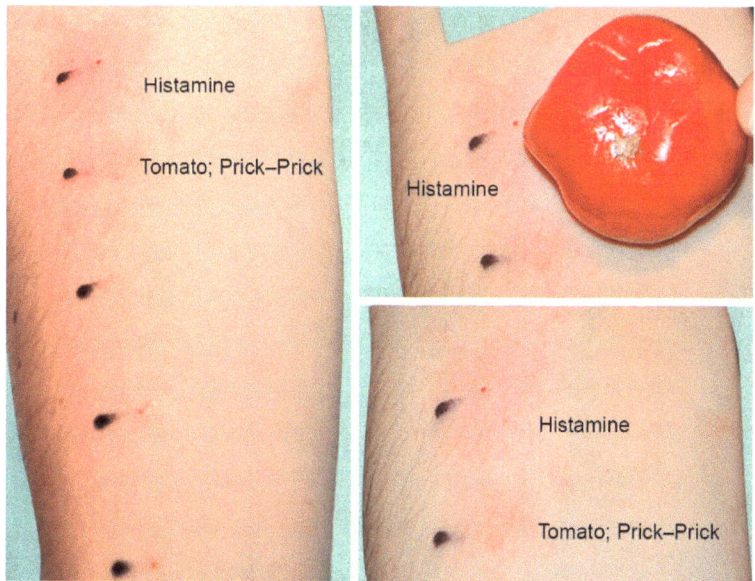

Fig. 3.1: Prick by prick positive by tomato, this agent was responsible of immediate erythema and evanescent wheals, chronic occupational exposure induced eczema.
Source: Hospital del Mar, IMIM.

showing both hives and eczema. Following the immediate reactions more chronic manifestations as eczema or dermatitis can be present during days and even weeks if the exposure with the responsible agent is maintained.

Based in an accurate anamnesis and physical examination (including occupational history) the disease diagnosis is easily performed. Nevertheless the identification of the responsible agents is necessary as preventive measures are based on its avoidance.[34] The knowledge of the specific diagnostic methods is crucial (Figs. 3.1 and 3.2).

Diagnostic Methods and Provocation Test

To make a correct diagnosis of ICSR, it is essential to have a complete clinical history, full physical examination and skin testing with suspected substances. Contact urticaria can be difficult to evaluate, because patients with CUS stage 1 or 2, they go to the medical advice when symptoms are no present or were modified by different treatments. In the same way, patients with stage 3 or 4 are quickly evaluated and usually receive urgent medical care, without being able to detect the causal agent. On the other hand, often is difficult to distinguish a simple skin irritation from CoU reaction. For this reason, is important an appropriate use of diagnostic test and their correct interpretation.

All in vitro test results should be evaluated alongside the clinical history, since allergen sensitization does not necessarily imply clinical responsiveness. In general, molecular diagnosis provide us specificity in the diagnosis, however, to have enough diagnostic sensitivity skin prick test or specific IgE with whole standardized extracts are required.[35]

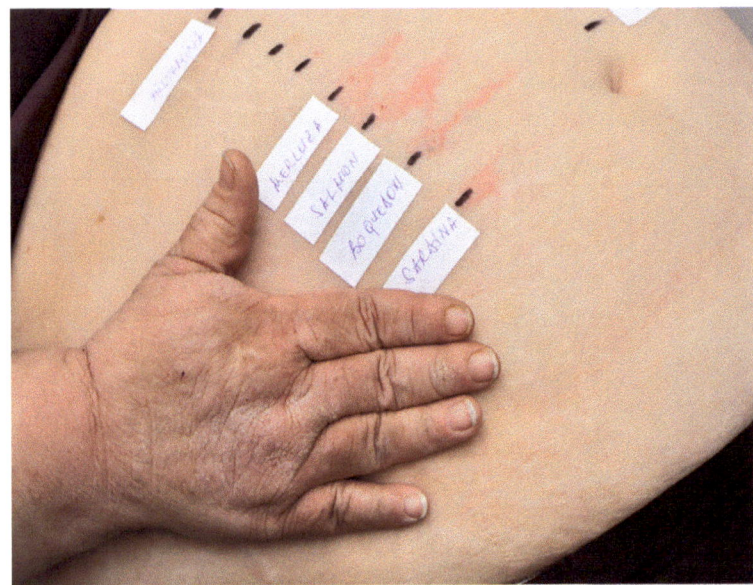

Fig. 3.2: Chronic eczema induced by chronic exposure to different types of fish to which an immediate positive prick by prick could be demonstrated; hake, salmon, anchovy and sardine.
Source: Hospital del Mar, IMIM.

The main role of tests to CoU diagnostic is identifying hypersensitivity type 1. Skin provocation tests for CoU are simple, quick and inexpensive. They are several in vivo types of tests (open test, closed chamber, scratch and scratch-patch test), but the simplest cutaneous provocation test for ICoU, NICoU and immediate contact dermatitis as PCD is the "open test".[36]

In the open test, the suspect substance (cosmetic, fruit, etc.) is applied onto normal skin area 3×3 cm^2 on upper arm. Reading is observed up to 1 hour and evaluated at 20 minutes, 40 minutes, and 60 minutes for erythema and edema.[37] The grading for erythema and edema is simple (+ weak, ++ moderate, +++ strong).[38] ICoU reaction usually appears after 15–20 minutes and often control site reaction is negative, being the NICoU one long lasting within 45–60 minutes, with control site reactions is mostly positive.[39] Immediate testing can also elicit non-urticarial reactions vesicular reactions as described in detail by Hjorth and Roed-Petersen in 1976 in a series of food handlers. They reported that open testing of incriminated foods on areas of the hands and fingers previously affected with dermatitis caused urticarial reactions in some patients, but others developed acute eruption of vesicles within 30 minutes.[10]

It is important to consider possible false negatives, as it happens with the use of nonsteroidal anti-inflammatory drugs and antihistamines. When the open test results are negative, "skin prick testing" (SPT) is often the method of choice for this type of reactions. Correctly used, the SPT has good sensitivity and specificity for detection of allergen-specific IgE and in some cases, its sensitivity may exceed that of in vitro assays. The results are available almost immediately, and it is usually less costly than in vitro testing. However, healthcare personnel who undertake SPT require skill and expertise, as correct technique is important.[40] In addition, the results are highly dependent on the allergen extract used. Skin prick test with fresh material or commercial reagents is the gold standard. The principle of the prick test relies on bringing a small volume of allergen (approximately 5–10 nL) into contact with mast cells by puncturing the skin with a lancet. When a prick by prick is done, with the same lancet the fresh material is pricked and immediately after the skin is punctured. A positive reaction elicited is assessed after 15–20 minutes compared with the positive control (histamine hydrochloride) and the negative control (sodium chloride). Flare is considered neuronal mediated and papule due to histamine release.[41]

TREATMENT

Contact urticaria syndrome, CoU, and PCD are conditions developed after immediate contact with different substances and allergens. The importance of studying and treating these reactions becomes relevant in the occupational setting, where CoU can account for 5–10% of occupational skin diseases,[42] with significant impact on the quality of life of workers and affecting laboral performance.[43]

The treatment for CUS is similar to other diseases triggered by hypersensitive type I reactions, being treated by prevention and antihistamines, in order to avoid mast cell's degranulation. Identifying and treating the cause of reaction is the most important measure, because the patient should be advised to avoid those allergens or substances, and their possible cross-reactions.

Given the safety profiles of antihistamines, those of second-generation should be of choice for the first-line treatment for urticaria. If it is necessary, higher doses of antihistamine can be used. When dermatitis is present, topical corticosteroids would be useful. In the severe cases of CUS, the use of systemic corticosteroids and emergency unit management may be necessary.

CONCLUSION

Immediate skin reactions are common in dermatological practice but still are underdiagnosed. CUS is a complete syndrome involving skin and mucosae and with potential systemic manifestations. Main cutaneous manifestations are hives and/or eczema/dermatitis, according to the nature of the allergen or trigger factor. The list of agents is very long and increase based in the publications of new isolated cases or short series of cases. Nevertheless plants, foods, vegetables and cosmetics continue to be the most common agents responsible of CUS. The same patient may develop hives and dermatitis suggesting an underlying immune mechanism for PCD similar to atopic dermatitis that has not been still well defined. The identification of the responsible agent and prevention are the most important measures to manage these patients, acquiring vital relevance in occupational dermatoses. The knowledge of this syndrome will help to identify these patients, understanding the possible triggers and mechanism to approach to the different clinical manifestation perform the proper study and diagnosis, in view of preventive measures and clinical advice.[44]

REFERENCES

1. Aquino M, Mawhirt S, Fonacier L. Review of contact urticaria syndrome-evaluation to treatment. Curr Treat Options Allergy. 2015;2:365-80.
2. Bathia R, Alikhan A, Maibach HI. Contact urticaria: present scenario. Indian J Dermatol. 2009;54:264-8.
3. Maibach HI, Johnson HL. Contact urticaria syndrome: contact urticaria to diethyltoluamide (immediate type hypersensitivity). Arch Dermatol. 1975;111:726-30.
4. Ring J (Ed). Allergy in practice. New York: Springer; 2005.

5. Gimenez-Arnau A, Isaksson M. Clinical Diagnosis of Immediate Contact Skin Reactions. In: Gimenez-Arnau A, Maibach H (Eds). Contact Urticaria Syndrome (1st edition). Switzerland: Springer International Publishing; 2018. p. 45.
6. Gimenez-Arnau A, Maibach HI. Contact urticarial syndrome. Florida: Taylor and Francis Group, LLC; 2015.
7. Wakelin SH. Contact Urticaria. Clin Exp Dermatol. 2001;26:132-6.
8. Maibach HI. Immediate hypersensitivity in hand dermatitis: role of food contact dermatitis. Arch Dermatol. 1976;112:1289-91.
9. Hannuksela M. Atopic contact dermatitis. Contact Derm. 1980;6:30.
10. Hjorth N, Roed-Petersen J. Occupational protein contact dermatitis in food handlers. Contact Derm. 1976;2:28-42.
11. Doutre MS. Occupational contact urticaria and protein contact dermatitis. Eur J Dermatol. 2005;15:419-24.
12. Gimenez-Arnau A, Maurer M, De la Cuadra J, et al. Immediate contact skin reactions, an update of contact urticaria, contact urticaria syndrome and protein contact dermatitis—"a never ending story". Eur J Dermatol. 2010;20:552-62.
13. Alfonso JH, Bauer A, Bensefa-Colas L, et al. Minimum standards on prevention, diagnosis and treatment of occupational and work-related skin diseases in Europe—position paper of the COST action StanDerm (TD 1206). J Eur Acad Dermatol Venearol. 2017;31:31-43.
14. Barbaud A, Poreaux C, Penven E, et al. Occupational protein contact dermatitis. Eur J Dermatol. 2015;25:527-34.
15. Lucaks J, Schliemann S, Elsner P. Occupational contact urticaria caused by food: a systemic clinical review. Contact Derm. 2016;75:195-204.
16. Vester L, Thyssen JP, Menne T, et al. Occupational food-related hand dermatoses seen over a 10-year period. Contact Dermatitis. 2012;66:264-70.
17. Fischer AA. Allergic contact urticaria of the hands due to seafood in food handlers. Cutis. 1988;42:388-9.
18. Gimenez-Arnau A, Isaksson M. Clinical Diagnosis of Immediate Contact Skin Reactions. In: Gimenez-Arnau A, Maibach H (Eds). Contact Urticaria Syndrome (1st edition). Switzerland: Springer International Publishing; 2018. p. 52.
19. Harvell J, Bason M, Maibach H. Contact urticarial and its mechanisms. Food Chem Toxicol. 1994;32:103-12.
20. Kligman AM. Dimethyl sulphoxide I and II. J Am Med Assoc. 1965;193:796-804,923-8.
21. Johansson J, Lahti A. Topical nonsteroidal anti-inflammatory drugs inhibit non-immunological immediate contact reactions. Contact Dermatitis. 1988;19:161-5.
22. Lahti A, Vaananen A, Kokkonen EL, et al. Acetylsalicylic acid inhibits non-immunologic contact urticaria. Contact Dermatitis. 1987;16:133-5.
23. Lahti A, Oikarinen A, Viinikka L, et al. Prostaglandins in contact urticaria induced by benzoic acid. Acta Dermatol Venereol (Stockh). 1983;63:425-7.
24. Amaro C, Goossens A. Immunological occupational contact urticaria and contact dermatitis from proteins: a review. Contact Dermatitis. 2008;58:67-75.
25. Kanerva L, Estlander T. Immediate and delayed skin allergy from cow dander. Am J Contact Dermat. 1997;8:167-9.
26. Conde-Salazar L, Gonzalez MA, Guimaraens D. Type I and Type IV sensitization to Anisakis simplex in 2 patients with hand eczema. Contact Dermatitis. 2002;46:361.
27. Garssen J, Vandebriel RJ, Kimber I, et al. Hypersensitivity reactions: definition, basic mechanics and localizations. In: Vos JG, Younes M, Smith E (Eds). Allergic Hypersensitivities Induced by Chemicals, Recommendations for Prevention. Boca Raton: CRC Press; 1996. pp. 19-58.
28. Von Krogh G, Maibach HI. The contact urticarial syndrome: An update review. J Am Acad Dermatol. 1981;5:328-42.

29. Gimenez-Arnau A, Isaksson M. Clinical Diagnosis of Immediate Contact Skin Reactions. In: Gimenez-Arnau A, Maibach H (Eds). Contact Urticaria Syndrome (1st edition). Switzerland: Springer International Publishing; 2018. pp. 48-9.
30. Czarnetzki B. Chapter 2: Basic mechanism. In: Czarnetzki MB (Ed). Urticaria. Berlin: Springer; 1986. pp. 5-25.
31. Zuberbier T, Aberer W, Asero R, et al. The EAACI/GA^{2}LEN/EDF/WAO guideline for the definition, classification, diagnosis and management of urticaria. Allergy. 2018;73:1393-414.
32. Gimenez-Arnau A, Isaksson M. Clinical Diagnosis of Immediate Contact Skin Reactions. In: Gimenez-Arnau A, Maibach H (Eds). Contact Urticaria Syndrome (1st edition). Switzerland: Springer International Publishing; 2018. p. 46.
33. Gimenez-Arnau A, Isaksson M. Clinical Diagnosis of Immediate Contact Skin Reactions. In: Gimenez-Arnau A, Maibach H (Eds). Contact Urticaria Syndrome (1st edition). Switzerland: Springer International Publishing; 2018. p. 49.
34. McFadden J. Inmunologic contact urticaria. Inmunol Allergy Clin N Am. 2014;34:157-67.
35. Sastre J. Molecular diagnosis in allergy. Clin Exp Allergy. 2010;40:1442-60.
36. Haustein UF Anaphylactic shock and contact urticaria after patch test with professional allergens. Allergie Immunol. 1976;22:349-52.
37. Amin S, Maibach HI. Inmunologic contact urticarial definition. Chapter 2. In: Amin S, Lahti A, Maibach HI (Eds). Contact urticarial syndrome. Boca Raton: CRC Press; 1997. pp. 11-26.
38. Amin S, Laverma A, Maibach HI. Diagnostic tests in dermatology. In: Maibach HI (Ed). Toxicology of skin. Philadelphia: Taylor and Francis; 2001. pp. 389-9.
39. Maucher OM. Anaphylaktische Reaktionen beim Epicutantest. Hautarzt. 1972;23:139-40.
40. Van Kampen V, deBlay F, Folleti I, et al. EAACI position paper: skin prick testing in the diagnosis of occupational type I allergies. Allergy. 2013;68:580-4.
41. Heinzerling L, Mari A, Bergmann K-C. The skin prick test – European standards. Clin Transl Allergy. 2013;3:3-10
42. Deza G, Gimenez-Arnau A. Management and treatment of contact urticaria syndrome. In: Gimenez-Arnau A, Maibach H (Eds). Contact Urticaria Syndrome (1st edition). Switzerland: Springer International Publishing; 2018. p. 161.
43. Bourrain JL. Occupational Contact Urticaria. Clin Rev Allergy Immunol. 2006;30:39-46.
44. Zuberbier T, Asero R, Bindslev-Jensen C, et al. EAACI/GA^{2}LEN/EDF guideline: management of urticaria. Allergy. 2009;64:1427-43.

CHAPTER 4

Chronic Inducible Urticaria

Andaç Salman, Ana M Giménez-Arnau

INTRODUCTION

Chronic inducible urticarias (CIndUs) are classified under the chronic urticaria which is defined by the occurrence of wheals, angioedema or both for at least 6 weeks.[1] The occurrence of wheals and/or angioedema in CIndUs requires the presence of a specific trigger. The CIndUs are further divided into physical urticaria and other inducible urticaria depending on the eliciting factors (Table 4.1).[2-4] Although generalized skin lesions or systemic symptoms may occur, the lesions are often localized to the skin in contact to the specific trigger. The CIndUs may coexist with chronic spontaneous urticaria (CSU) or more than one type of CIndU may be present in the same individual.[3] In one series, 36.3% of the patients were reported to have at least one positive provocation test result. The most common forms of CIndUs coexisting with CSU are symptomatic dermographism (SD) and delayed pressure urticaria (DPU).[5]

The diagnosis of CIndUs requires a thorough patient history to identify possible eliciting factors. In any patient with a history suggesting a triggering factor, the standardized provocation tests should be performed.[3]

Table 4.1: Classification and triggering factors of chronic inducible urticarias (CIndUs).

	Synonyms	Triggering factors
Physical		
Symptomatic dermographism	Urticaria factitia, dermographic urticaria	Shearing forces on the skin
Cold urticaria	Acquired cold urticaria, cold contact urticaria	Contact cooling of the skin with cool air, liquid or solid objects
Heat urticaria	Heat contact urticaria	Contact heating of the skin
Delayed pressure urticaria	Pressure urticaria	Sustained pressure applied to the skin
Solar urticaria		Exposure to sunlight
Vibratory angioedema		Exposure to vibration
Other CIndUs		
Cholinergic urticaria		Exercise or passive warming
Aquagenic urticaria		Any source of hot or cold water

CHRONIC INDUCIBLE URTICARIAS DIAGNOSTIC PROVOCATION TESTS AND DISEASE CONTROL

The caution is advised during provocation tests, because in patients with severe CIndUs systemic reactions ranging from dizziness, diarrhea to anaphylactic shock may occur. Experienced and trained physicians in these conditions should perform the provocation tests and emergency treatment equipment should be available.

Discontinuation of the antihistamines (3 days before testing) and glucocorticoids (at least 7 days before testing) and choosing a test site which was not affected for at least 24 hours are recommended to avoid false negative test results.[3]

The provocation testing allows identifying the eliciting factor and determining the trigger thresholds. Threshold assessment is recommended because it is very helpful for the proper counseling of the patients and monitoring the treatment response. The results of the provocation tests should be evaluated 10 minutes after testing except for DPU in which the lesions may develop up to 6 hours after provocation. The details for standardized provocation and threshold testing for CIndUs are provided in Tables 4.2 and 4.3.[3] A recent study have reported a high negative predictive value but a low predictive value of provocation testing in patients with cold, heat and DPU.[6] Therefore in some patients with a highly suggestive history of such CIndUs, the diagnosis cannot be certified with the standardized provocation tests. In those cases, it is

Table 4.2: Provocation tests for chronic inducible urticarias (CIndUs).

CIndU	Test site	Methods	Reading time after testing	Positive test
Symptomatic dermographism	Volar forearm or upper back	Moderate stroking with a smooth blunt object, dermographometer (36 g/mm^2), FricTest	10 min	Pruritic wheal
Cold urticaria	Volar forearm	Ice cubes in a plastic bag, cold water baths, TempTest (4–44°C) for 5 min	10 min	Wheal
Heat urticaria	Volar forearm	Metal or glass cylinders filled with hot water, hot water baths, TempTest (44–4°C) for 5 min	10 min	Wheal
Delayed pressure urticaria	Shoulder/ upper back/ thighs/volar forearm	Suspension of weights over shoulder (7 kg, shoulder strap width: 3 cm) for 15 min OR weighted rods (1.5 cm diameter: 2.5 kg; or 6.5 cm diameter: 5 kg) for 15 min. OR dermographometer (100 g/mm^2 for 70 sec)	6 h	Angioedema and erythema
Solar urticaria	Buttocks	UVA 6 J/cm^2 AND UVB 60 mJ/cm^2 and visible light (slide projector)	10 min	Wheal
Vibratory angioedema	Volar forearm	Vortex vibrator for 5 min, at 1,000 rpm	10 min	Angioedema or wheal
Cholinergic urticaria	N/A	Exercise with stationary bike or treadmill (for 30 min, increase pulse rate by 3 BPM) *if positive:* Passive warming with hot baths (42°C bath for 15 min, until body temperature has increased 1°C or more) Pulse-controlled ergometry	Throughout the test and 10 min	Wheals
Aquagenic urticaria	Trunk	A compress or a towel soaked with water at 35–37°C or physiologic saline for 40 min or less	10 min	Wheal

Table 4.3: Threshold testing for chronic inducible urticarias (CIndUs).[3]

CIndU	Test site	Methods	Reading time after testing	Threshold
Symptomatic dermographism	Volar forearm or upper back	Dermographometer, FricTest	10 min	Lowest trigger strength (pin size for FricTest and strength in g/mm^2 for dermographometer) that causes a pruritic wheal
Cold urticaria	Volar forearm	TempTest 4® (4–44°C) for 5 min	10 min	Highest temperature inducing a wheal *Stimulation time threshold (shortest duration of cold exposure to induce a wheal) may also be assessed.
Heat urticaria	Volar forearm	TempTest 4® (44–°C) for 5 min	10 min	Lowest temperature inducing a wheal *Stimulation time threshold (shortest duration of heat exposure to induce a wheal) may also be assessed.
Delayed pressure urticaria	Volar forearm (rods) or upper back (dermographometer)	Weighted rods or dermographometer for 15 min	6 h	Rod with lowest weight (1-2-3-4-5 kg) causing angioedema and erythema
Solar urticaria	Buttocks	UVA/UVB irradiation	10 min	Lowest dose of irradiation (UVA: 2.4, 3.3, 4.2, 5.1, 6 J/cm^2; UVB: 24, 33, 42, 51, 60 mJ/cm^2) causing a wheal response

Source: Adapted from Magerl M, Altrichter S, Borzova E, et al. The definition, diagnostic testing, and management of chronic inducible urticarias—The EAACI/GA²LEN/EDF/UNEV consensus recommendations 2016 update and revision. Allergy. 2016;71:780-802.

useful to adapt the recommended test to the clinical history of the patients, e.g. in localized cold urticaria (ColdU) or atypical forms of ColdU. The provocation test and the assessment of baseline thresholds help to assess the benefits of the treatment.

Actually the use of the validated patient report outcome urticaria control test (UCT) is recommended to be used in routine clinical practice for assessing the disease control.[7]

BASIS OF CHRONIC INDUCIBLE URTICARIAS MANAGEMENT

Considering the severe impact on quality of life and possible systemic reactions, early diagnosis and treatment are essential. The avoidance of the trigger is the mainstay of treatment and usually very challenging for the most of the patients. In addition to trigger avoidance, symptomatic treatment options include H1 antihistamines, leukotriene receptor antagonists, omalizumab or cyclosporine.[3,8,9] Treatment alternatives including immunomodulatory drugs and desensitization for each type of CIndU is addressed in detail in Table 4.4.

Table 4.4: Treatment options for chronic inducible urticarias (CIndUs).

CIndU	Treatment options		
	Level of evidence A	Level of evidence B	Level of evidence C
Symptomatic dermographism	H1 antihistamines	Phototherapy Cyclosporine Omalizumab	
Cold urticaria	H1 antihistamines Omalizumab	Desensitization Antibiotics	Cyclosporine Danazol Zafirlukast Etanercept Anakinra
Heat urticaria			H1 antihistamines Omalizumab Desensitization
Delayed pressure urticaria	H1 antihistamines and/or leukotriene antagonists	Omalizumab Sulfasalazine Dapsone Theophylline	Oral coumarins Chloroquine Anti-TNF-alpha Tranexamic acid
Solar urticaria	H1 antihistamines	Omalizumab H1 antihistamines and/or leukotriene antagonists Phototherapy Intravenous immunoglobulins Alpha-MSH hormone analog	Plasmapheresis Cyclosporine
Vibratory angioedema			H1 antihistamines Amitriptyline and bromazepam Ketotifen
Cholinergic urticaria	H1 antihistamines Combination of H1 and H2 antihistamines Danazol	Desensitization with autologous sweat Omalizumab	Methanthelinium bromide Botulinum toxin Surgical ganglion blokage Ketotifen Scopolamine Beta blockers
Aquagenic urticaria			Phototherapy and antihistamines H1 antihistamines Barrier cream

Level of evidence A: double-blinded controlled studies; Level of evidence B: case series or uncontrolled studies with more than 5 patients; Level of evidence C: case reports or small case series.[3]

CHRONIC INDUCIBLE URTICARIAS PATHOGENESIS

The symptoms of CIndUs are largely caused by the activation and degranulation of mast cells followed by the release of proinflammatory cytokines.[10] Also the efficacy of anti-immunoglubulin (anti-IgE) treatment in various forms of CIndUs suggests a role for IgE in the activation of mast cells through the FcεIgE receptor.[11] Moreover, increased serum levels of IgE in patients with CIndUs and passive transfer of the disease by transferring the serum of the patients are in support with the role of IgE.[12-14]

In cholinergic urticaria (CholU) increased histamine levels, acetylcholine, sweat allergy, associated serum factors, poral occlusion, hypohidrosis/anhidrosis are suggested to take part in the pathogenesis.[15] In aquagenic urticaria (AU), the research have demonstrated the role of sudden changes in osmotic pressure around the hair follicles[16] and suggest that water-soluble antigens in the epidermis penetrating the skin are responsible of the water-induced erythema and wheals.[17,18] In solar urticaria, the role of skin or serum molecules turning into photoallergens with specific wavelengths has been investigated.[19]

Although various possible eliciting factors, e.g. infections have been proposed for different forms of CIndUs, the exact pathophysiology still remains to be understood.

SYMPTOMATIC DERMOGRAPHISM

Symptomatic dermographism, or urticaria factitia, dermographic urticaria, is the most frequent type of CIndU.[3]

Epidemiology

The frequency of SD is estimated to be 1–5% in the general population.[3] SD usually has a chronic course with a mean duration of disease of approximately 6 years.[8]

Clinical Features

Development of itchy wheals occur due to shearing forces on the skin which may be caused by rubbing, scratching or scrubbing.[3,8] The differential diagnosis includes simple dermographism, which is characterized by the development of erythema or wheals without pruritus.

Diagnosis

The diagnosis of the SD requires a provocation test which can be performed either with a blunt object or instruments such as dermographometer and FricTest[3] (Fig. 4.1).

A smooth blunt object (a pen or a wooden tongue spatula) should be applied perpendicularly to the skin creating a light pressure on the volar forearm or upper back. The test site should be intact and free of any inflammation or infection. The test site should be assessed within 10 minutes of provocation and a pruritic wheal is considered positive. Erythema or just wheal formation without pruritus favors simple dermographism.

Another provocation method for SD is the use of a calibrated dermographometer, which also enables physician to assess the trigger threshold. Symptomatic dermographism is diagnosed if the wheal appears at a pressure less than or equal to 36 g/cm^2.[20] FricTest (MOXIE GmbH, Berlin, *info@moxie-gmbh.de* or *www.moxie-gmbh.de*) is new device validated for the diagnosis of SD. It has four plastic tips with the same diameter of 3 mm and different lengths ranging from 3 mm to 4.5 mm. It is applied perpendicular to the volar forearm skin. Owing to its four tips

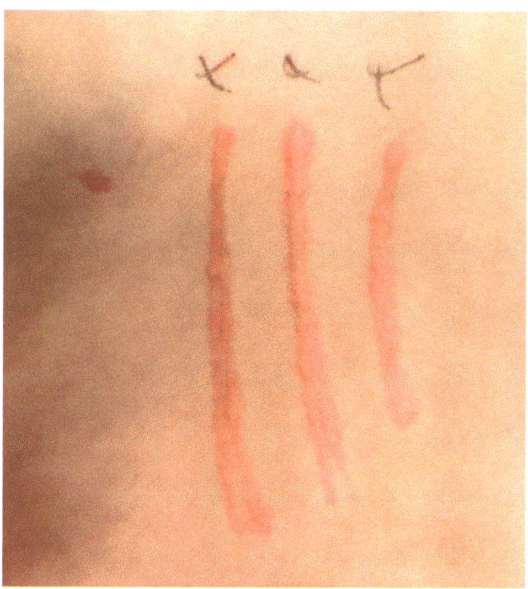

Fig. 4.1: Symptomatic dermographism assessed by dermographometer and FricTest®.
Source: Hospital del Mar, IMIM.

with different lengths, the shearing forces are applied to the skin in a graded manner, thus the trigger threshold can be determined. The development of a pruritic wheal more than or equal to 3 mm width within 10 minutes of provocation is considered positive.[3]

Treatment

Besides trigger avoidance, the first-line treatment for SD is nonsedating second-generation H1 antihistamines.[9] In patients with inadequate symptom control, the H1 antihistamine doses can be increased up to four-fold. The third-line treatment alternative is omalizumab.[21,22] In addition, the use of phototherapy modalities may be of benefit in some patients as the literature data suggests.[3,9,23]

COLD URTICARIA

Cold urticaria, also known as acquired cold urticaria (ACU), cold contact urticaria or urticaria a frigore is characterized by the development of wheals and flare skin type reactions and angioedema after contact cooling of the skin by cold air, liquids or solids[3] (Fig. 4.2).

Epidemiology

It is the second most common type of physical urticaria.[3] It usually affects young adults with a slight female predominance. Its annual incidence is estimated to be 0.05%.[24] In a cohort study 5- and 10-year resolution rates of ColdU were 17.9% and 24.5%, respectively.[25]

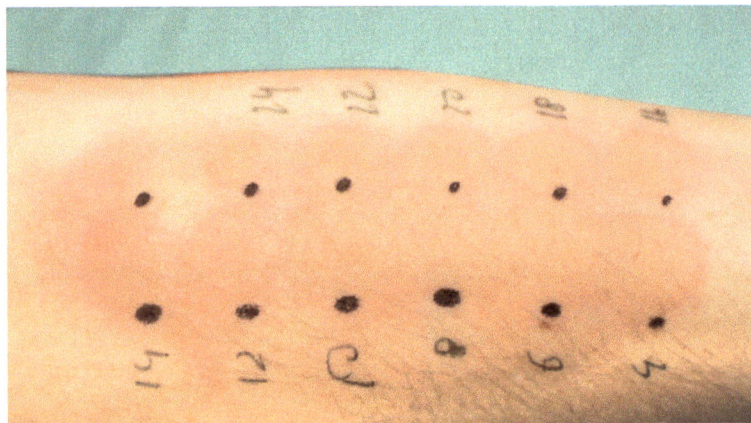

Fig. 4.2: Critical temperature threshold in a patient with severe cold urticaria (ColdU), CTT 24°C.
Source: Hospital del Mar, IMIM.

Clinical Features

The symptoms may occur within minutes following the contact with cold air, liquids or solid objects.[3] Acquired cold urticaria may be idiopathic (primary) or secondary to cryoproteinemia, lymphoproliferative diseases, viral infections including hepatitis B, C and infectious mononucleosis. Thus, the possible underlying causes should be ruled out. The urticarial lesions might be localized, generalized or associated with severe systemic reactions including hypotension and respiratory distress.[3,24,26,27] Up to 19% of patients with ColdU have reported life-threatening reactions. The most common trigger of severe systemic reactions is aquatic activities in cold water. According with Mlynek A et al.[28] the mean temperature capable to induce ACU is 17 ± 6°C (range 4–27°C). Based in a Likert scale we could classify ACU as mild (12.3 ± 8°C), moderate (18.6 ± 7.1°C), and severe (2.0 ± 2.5°C). The patients with severe disease are expected to have longer duration of disease and worse response to treatment with no sedating H1 antihistamines.[24]

The patients with ColdU and a negative provocation test are defined as atypical ACU. An earlier study has reported an increased frequency of systemic reactions in such patients, but the latter studies have failed to demonstrate such relation.[24,26]

Higher rates of atypical ACU along with lower likelihood of achieving a complete symptom resolution was observed in patients with the onset of symptoms during childhood ($p < 0.05$). In patients with atypical ACU, shorter disease duration and lower doses of antihistamines required for achieving disease control were detected ($p < 0.05$). Age at disease onset, symptom severity and ColdU thresholds values were found to be related with longer disease evolution ($p < 0.05$).[19]

Diagnosis

Provocation testing should be performed on the volar forearm skin. Traditional methods include ice cube test and cold water baths.[3] In case of ice cube test, ice cubes in a plastic bag should be used to avoid direct water contact and exclude AU. Critical stimulation time threshold (CsTT) can be assessed by different time exposure to the ice cube. A CsTT less than 3 minutes founded to be

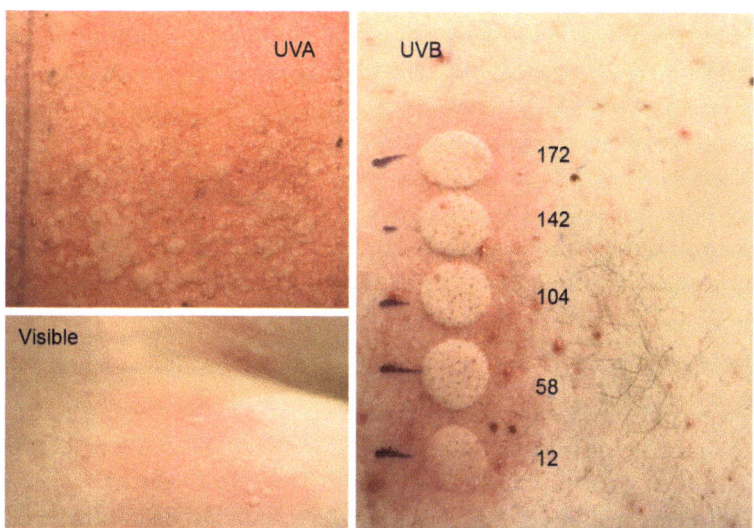

Fig. 4.3: Solar urticaria (SU), induced by ultraviolet A (UVA) and visible light.
Source: Hospital del Mar, IMIM.

associated with higher disease severity compared with more than 3 minutes.[26] Cold water bath can be used, when the ice cube is negative but caution is warranted as it may induce systemic reactions. Another method for the provocation and trigger threshold test is TempTest4® (Courage and Khazaka, Köln, Germany) which is a Peltier element-based device.[29] It allows performing provocation tests for cold and heat by applying a continuous temperature gradient from 4°C to 44°C. The temperature and stimulation time thresholds can also be determined with TempTest3® (Fig. 4.3). The standardized time for cold provocation testing is 5 minutes. But it can be adjusted to shorter or longer times for patients who are very sensitive or patients with a positive history but without wheals after standard testing, respectively. The test sites should be evaluated 10 minutes after provocation. For patients with a positive provocation test, stimulation time and temperature threshold testing are recommended. The threshold testing are useful for patient counseling, evaluating the disease severity and monitoring the efficacy of treatment.[3,30,31]

Treatment

The first-line treatment for ColdU is nonsedating H1 antihistamines.[3,9,32] However, high doses of H1 antihistamines might be required for symptom control in many patients. Recently, the results of a randomized placebo-controlled study have shown that omalizumab in doses of 150 mg and 300 mg is effective and well-tolerated in patients with ColdU.[33] Other treatment options reported in the literature are cyclosporine, antibiotic treatment (doxycycline or penicillin) and cold desensitization.[34-37] Danazol, anakinra, etanercept, and reslizumab (anti-interleukin-5) have also been reported to be effective in anecdotal reports.[38,39] In addition, prescription of epinephrine autoinjectors for patients who had episodes of cold-induced anaphylaxis and angioedema affecting oropharynx is recommended by some authors.[8,40]

HEAT URTICARIA

Heat urticaria (HU), or heat contact urticaria, is a very rare condition characterized by the occurrence of wheals upon contact with heat.[3]

Epidemiology

It is very rare form of CIndUs.[3] A recent analysis of the published cases revealed 60 patients in the literature. The most of the patients were female and the age of onset of the HU was 34.4 years.[41]

Clinical Features

The wheals develop within minutes of exposure to heat source. Warm baths, hot air and exposure to sun are the most common triggers. Two clinical types of HU were described: (1) immediate HU and (2) delayed HU. Most of the patients had immediate type HU with wheal developing within minutes and resolving within 1–3 hours. On the other hand, in delayed type HU, the wheal/angioedema response occurs 30 minutes to 2 hours after exposure to heat and they resolve within 12-14 hours.[41] In some patients with immediate HU generalized lesions and systemic symptoms including wheezing, syncope episodes may also be seen. Itching is the most frequent symptom in patients with HU although burning sensation was also reported in delayed HU.[41] It should be differentiated from solar urticaria and CholU through the standardized provocation tests.

Diagnosis

Heat provocation testing might be performed using metal/glass cylinders filled with hot water, hot water baths or TempTest4®. Although the standard testing consists of applying heat (at temperatures up to 44ªC) for 5 minutes to the skin of the volar forearm, time and temperature adjustments might be done for some patients. The test site should be evaluated 10 minutes after provocation.[3] Similarly with the ColdU, stimulation time and temperature threshold can be assessed in patients with a positive provocation testing.[23]

Treatment

Because the condition is very rare, the treatment options reported are limited in the literature. Heat desensitization provided a complete response in 60% of the patients. No sedating H1 antihistamines at standard and high doses was effective but full control of symptoms were not common.[41] Omalizumab led to complete remission in three patients.[23,41,42] Colchicine, chloroquine, montelukast, and cyclosporine failed to show any benefit in case reports.[41]

DELAYED PRESSURE URTICARIA

Delayed pressure urticaria is characterized by the development of wheals/angioedema upon sustained pressure applied to the skin.[3]

Epidemiology

Although the occurrence of DPU as a primary CIndU is rare, its coexistence with CSU is common, affecting between 6.7% and 17% of patients with CSU.[5,43-45]

Clinical Features

The development of the lesions usually takes 6–8 hours (ranging from 30 minutes to 12 hours) and they may persist up to 72 hours. Unlike the other forms of CIndUs, the lesions are associated with burning or pain rather than itching. The clinical differential diagnosis includes SD in which the lesions develop immediately after physical stimulus.[3]

Diagnosis

The provocation testing is done by application of a sustained pressure to the skin. There are several methods including suspension of weights over the shoulder, the application of rods or dermographometer.[20] The weights and rod diameters vary greatly in the literature. The dermographometer is applied for 70 seconds with a pressure of 100 g/mm^2. The test response should be assessed 6 hours after the provocation testing by the physician or the patient.[3,46]

Treatment

The patients with DPU should avoid sustained pressure to the skin such as tight clothing. In addition to standard and higher doses of H1 antihistamines; omalizumab was reported to effective in 3 patients with DPU.[3,9,43] Moreover, dapsone and sulfasalazine have been reported to be effective in large series of patients with DPU.[47,48] Other treatment alternatives are montelukast, colchicine, dapsone, sulfasalazine, escitalopram, anti-TNF, and theophylline.[3,9,49,50]

SOLAR URTICARIA

Solar urticaria (SU) is an idiopathic photodermatosis and a form of CIndU characterized by the development of wheals within minutes following exposure to sunlight.[3,51]

Epidemiology

It is rare condition affecting females more frequently. The mean age of the patients ranged from 29.8 years to 37.9 years in different series.[51,52]

Clinical Features

The urticarial lesions and erythema appear within minutes after exposure to the sun and mostly involve sun-exposed areas. The skin covered with thin clothing may also be affected. Delayed onset of symptoms and systemic anaphylactic reactions were also reported.[51] The most commonly involved action spectrum was visible light followed by ultraviolet A (UVA) and ultraviolet B (UVB).[51,52] The differential diagnosis includes polymorphous light eruption, which is characterized with development of papular, and papulovesicular lesions within hours of sun exposure and persisting up to a few weeks.

Diagnosis

The diagnosis is made based on history and provocation testing. Discontinuation of the sunscreen and photosensitizing medications before testing is recommended. Solar simulators or monochromator might be used for provocation and the assessment of the minimal urticarial dose (MUD). A slide projector can be used for provocation with visible light. The recommended test site is the buttock and photoprovocation with UVA (6 J/cm^2), UVB (60 mJ/cm^2) and visible light should be performed separately. Urticarial response at the test site within 10 minutes is considered positive. Threshold testing with varying dose of the radiation might be helpful in determining disease severity and response to therapy.[2,3]

Treatment

In addition to strict use of sunscreens, the most frequently used treatment is nonsedating H1 antihistamines.[51] Recently, omalizumab was reported to provide complete clinical remission in patients with SU.[23,53,54] Desensitization, intravenous immunoglobulins, phototherapy modalities, cyclosporine, and afamelanotide have also been reported to be effective.[3,9,51]

VIBRATORY ANGIOEDEMA

Vibratory angioedema (VA) is characterized by an urticarial response to vibration.[3,55]

Epidemiology

Very rare.

Clinical Features

The wheals develop within minutes after exposure to vibration. Atypical forms of VA with delayed onset of lesions or familial forms have also been reported.[56-58]

Diagnosis

The provocation test can be performed using a laboratory vortex mixer. The forearm is held on the vortex mixer that is run between 780 rpm and 1,380 rpm for 5 minutes. The test site is assessed after 10 minutes and the increase of the circumference of the tested arm compared to pretest is considered a positive test.[3]

Treatment

In addition to avoidance of trigger, treatment options are limited to nonsedating H1 antihistamines.[9] Anti-IgE treatment with omalizumab failed to show benefit in one patient.[59]

CHOLINERGIC URTICARIA

Cholinergic urticaria is characterized with pinpoint sized wheal formation triggered by an increase in the core body temperature induced by exercise, emotional stress and hot baths.[3]

Epidemiology

It affect approximately 4–11.2% of the general population and 20% of the young adults.[3,15]

Clinical Features

The lesions are typically pinpoint sized wheals with surrounding erythema mostly affecting the trunk and extremities. The lesions may sometimes coalesce into larger plaques and usually resolve rapidly within 15–60 minutes.[3] Stinging and tingling sensation are more common than itching. The subjective symptoms usually cause a severe impairment in quality of life and recently the first CholU-specific quality of life instrument has been developed.[15,60]

Recently four subtypes of CholU have been proposed: conventional sweat-allergy type CholU, CholU with palpebral angioedema (CholU-PA), follicular-type CholU with a positive autologous serum skin test (ASST), and CholU with acquired anhidrosis and/or hypohidrosis.[15,61] Conventional sweat-allergy type CholU is caused by sweat allergy and can be diagnosed with a positive autologous sweat skin test (ASwST). CholU-PA is most seen in females and associated with a strong atopic predisposition. ASwST is frequently positive and periorbital angioedema is a distinguishing clinical feature. CholU with acquired anhidrosis and/or hypohidrosis shows a male predominance and always associated with hypo/anhidrosis.[15,62]

Another research has suggested that early-onset CholU (before 36 years of age) is more frequently associated with atopy whereas patients with late-onset CholU are usually female and more likely to have a shorter duration of disease and coexisting other forms of urticaria.[63] The association with atopy is frequent and those with atopic predisposition have more severe CholU.[64]

Severe CholU can even show anaphylaxis[65] but the differential diagnosis includes exercise-induced anaphylaxis which is induced with physical exercise. In contrast to CholU, the lesions are larger and start from the distal parts of the body. The provocation testing with physical exercise is positive, however passive warming test with hot bath is only positive in patients with CholU.[3]

Diagnosis

Provocation testing helps to confirm the diagnosis of CholU and exclude exercise-induced anaphylaxis. An exercise test with a treadmill or stationary bike should be done for 15 minutes or until the onset of symptoms. The typical eruption develops within 10 minutes after testing. A standardized protocol using a pulse-controlled ergometry has also been proposed recently.[3,66] Stop at a final maximum increase of 90 beats/min above the starting level at 30 minutes or at onset of whealing. The onset of sweating and whealing is recorded. In case of a positive exercise test, a passive warming test with hot bath should be performed to rule out exercise-induced anaphylaxis.

Treatment

In CholU with normal sweat function, the first-line treatment is nonsedating H1 antihistamines. In patients with no response updosing of H1 antihistamines, montelukast or omalizumab are recommended.[15] In patients with hypohidrotic CholU, nonsedating H1 antihistamines or in case of severe disease pulse steroid therapy might be of benefit.[15]

Successful use of scopolamine, propranolol, desensitization to sweat, and danazol have been reported in the literature.[9,15]

AQUAGENIC URTICARIA

Aquagenic urticaria is rare condition in which the contact with any source of hot or cold water provokes an urticarial response.[3]

Epidemiology

The AU is very rare with more than 50 cases reported in the literature. The prevalence is higher among females and the typical time of onset is during puberty or postpuberty.[67]

Clinical Features

The lesions are usually 1–2 mm in size, folliculocentric and develop within 30 minutes of exposure to water. They usually resolve within 30–60 minutes. The lesions mostly involve the trunk and upper proximal extremities.[3,67] Although it is mostly sporadic, familial cases have also been reported.[68] Systemic symptoms such as wheezing or dyspnea may occur albeit rare. The differential diagnosis includes aquagenic pruritus, CholU, ColdU, and HU. The latter three can be differentiated through careful provocation testing (see Table 4.3). The aquagenic pruritus is characterized with pruritus but no skin lesions following exposure to water. It is usually associated with hematological disorders such as polycythemia vera and often recalcitrant to AU treatment.[69]

Diagnosis

The provocation test is done with a compress or a towel soaked with water at 35–37°C or physiologic saline on the trunk. The towel or compress is applied to skin for 40 minutes or less if the patient reports pruritus and the wheals develop. The test area should be assessed within 10 minutes.[3]

Treatment

Besides the trigger avoidance, treatment options are limited to mostly to the use of H1 antihistamines. Other treatments as UV therapy, anticholinergic agents such as scopolamine (based on the cholinergic pathogenic theory) and barrier creams preventing water contact with skin show a very limited efficacy.[18,67,70]

Globally CIndUs shows specific distinctive clinical features, showing a lower gender rate female/male than CSU. Patients with CIndU are significantly younger than patients with CSU. Patients with CIndUs show less thyroid and psychiatric comorbidities and suffer less exacerbation due to acetylsalicylic acid (ASA) and nonsteroidal anti-inflammatory drugs (NSAIDs). The episodes of angioedema are more common in CSU. Finally, CIndUs commonly get control with second-generation antihistamines at licensed doses or up dosing them, although alternative treatments as new anti-IgE therapy or desensitization were used with success. Less frequents than CSU, the CIndUs impaired hardly the quality of life and require a good strategic management efficient and safe.

REFERENCES

1. Zuberbier T, Aberer W, Asero R, et al. The EAACI/GA^{2}LEN/EDF/WAO guideline for the definition, classification, diagnosis and management of urticaria. Allergy. 2018;73:1393-414. doi:10.1111/all.13397.
2. Magerl M, Borzova E, Giménez-Arnau A, et al. The definition and diagnostic testing of physical and cholinergic urticarias—EAACI/GA^{2}LEN/EDF/UNEV consensus panel recommendations. Allergy. 2009;64:1715-21.
3. Magerl M, Altrichter S, Borzova E, et al. The definition, diagnostic testing, and management of chronic inducible urticarias—The EAACI/GA^{2}LEN/EDF/UNEV consensus recommendations 2016 update and revision. Allergy. 2016;71:780-802.
4. Trevisonno J, Balram B, Netchiporouk E, et al. Physical urticaria: Review on classification, triggers and management with special focus on prevalence including a meta-analysis. Postgrad Med. 2015;127:565-70.
5. Sánchez J, Amaya E, Acevedo A, et al. Prevalence of inducible urticaria in patients with chronic spontaneous urticaria: Associated risk factors. J Allergy Clin Immunol Pract. 2017;5:464-70.
6. Holm JG, Agner T, Thomsen SF. Diagnostic properties of provocation tests for cold, heat, and delayed-pressure urticaria. Eur J Dermatol. 2017;27:406-8.
7. Weller K, Groffik A, Church MK, et al. Development and validation of the urticaria control test: a patient-reported outcome instrument for assessing urticaria control. J Allergy Clin Immunol. 2014;133:1365-72, 1372.e1-6.
8. Maurer M, Fluhr JW, Khan DA. How to approach chronic inducible urticaria. J Allergy Clin Immunol Pract. 2018;6:1119-30.
9. Dressler C, Werner RN, Eisert L, et al. Chronic inducible urticaria: A systematic review of treatment options. J Allergy Clin Immunol. 2018;141:1726-34.
10. Church MK, Kolkhir P, Metz M, et al. The role and relevance of mast cells in urticaria. Immunol Rev. 2018;282:232-47.
11. Maurer M, Metz M, Brehler R, et al. Omalizumab treatment in patients with chronic inducible urticaria: A systematic review of published evidence. J Allergy Clin Immunol. 2018;141:638-49.
12. Altrichter S, Peter HJ, Pisarevskaja D, et al. IgE mediated autoallergy against thyroid peroxidase—a novel pathomechanism of chronic spontaneous urticaria? PLoS One. 2011;6:e14794.
13. Houser DD, Arbesman CE, Ito K, et al. Cold urticaria: Immunologic studies. Am J Med. 1970;49:23-33.
14. Newcomb RW, Nelson H. Dermographia mediated by immunoglobulin E. Am J Med. 1973;54:174-80.
15. Fukunaga A, Washio K, Hatakeyama M, et al. Cholinergic urticaria: epidemiology, physiopathology, new categorization, and management. Clin Auton Res. 2018;28:103-13.
16. Tkach JR. Aquagenic urticaria. Cutis. 1981;28:454-63.
17. Czarnetzki BM, Breetholt KH, Traupe H. Evidence that water acts as a carrier for an epidermal antigen in aquagenic urticaria. J Am Acad Dermatol. 1986;15:623-7.
18. Gimenez-Arnau A, Serra-Baldrich E, Camarasa JG. Chronic aquagenic urticaria. Acta Derm Venereol. 1992;72:389.
19. Botto NC, Warshaw EM. Solar urticaria. J Am Acad Dermatol. 2008;59:909-20; quiz 921-2.
20. Lawlor F, Black AK. Delayed pressure urticaria. Immunol Allergy Clin North Am. 2004;24:247-58, vi-vii.
21. Maurer M, Metz M, Brehler R, et al. Omalizumab treatment in patients with chronic inducible urticaria: A systematic review of published evidence. J Allergy Clin Immunol. 2017;141:1-12.
22. Maurer M, Schütz A, Weller K, et al. Omalizumab is effective in symptomatic dermographism—results of a randomized placebo-controlled trial. J Allergy Clin Immunol. 2017;140:870-73.e5.
23. Maurer M, Metz M, Brehler R, et al. Omalizumab treatment in patients with chronic inducible urticaria: A systematic review of published evidence. J Allergy Clin Immunol. 2018;141:638-49.
24. Deza G, Brasileiro A, Bertolín-Colilla M, et al. Acquired cold urticaria: Clinical features, particular phenotypes, and disease course in a tertiary care center cohort. J Am Acad Dermatol. 2016;75:918-24.e2.

25. Jain SV, Mullins RJ. Cold urticaria: a 20-year follow-up study. J Eur Acad Dermatology Venereol. 2016;30:2066-71.
26. Wanderer AA, Grandel KE, Wasserman SI, et al. Clinical characteristics of cold-induced systemic reactions in acquired cold urticaria syndromes: Recommendations for prevention of this complication and a proposal for a diagnostic classification of cold urticaria. J Allergy Clin Immunol. 1986;78:417-23.
27. Mathelier-Fusade P, Aïssaoui M, Bakhos D, et al. Clinical predictive factors of severity in cold urticaria. Arch Dermatol. 1998;134:106-7.
28. Młynek A, Magerl M, Siebenhaar F, et al. Results and relevance of critical temperature threshold testing in patients with acquired cold urticaria. Br J Dermatol. 2010;162:198-200.
29. Siebenhaar F, Staubach P, Metz M, et al. Peltier effect-based temperature challenge: an improved method for diagnosing cold urticaria. J Allergy Clin Immunol. 2004;114:1224-5.
30. Neittaanmäki H. Cold urticaria. J Am Acad Dermatol. 1985;13:636-44.
31. Martinez-Escala ME, Curto-Barredo L, Carnero L, et al. Temperature thresholds in assessment of the clinical course of acquired cold contact urticaria: a prospective observational one-year study. Acta Derm Venereol. 2015;95:278-82.
32. Abajian M, Curto-Barredo L, Krause K, et al. Rupatadine 20 mg and 40 mg are effective in reducing the symptoms of chronic cold urticaria. Acta Derm Venereol. 2016;96:56-9.
33. Metz M, Schütz A, Weller K, et al. Omalizumab is effective in cold urticaria—results of a randomized placebo-controlled trial. J Allergy Clin Immunol. 2017;140:864-67.e5.
34. Marsland AM, Beck MH. Cold urticaria responding to systemic ciclosporin. Br J Dermatol. 2003;149:214-5.
35. Liebeskind H, Schwarze G. Penicillin therapy in cold contact urticaria. Hautarzt. 1974;25:482-5.
36. Gorczyza M, Schoepke N, Krause K, et al. Patients with chronic cold urticaria may benefit from doxycycline therapy. Br J Dermatol. 2017;176:259-61.
37. Black AK, Sibbald RG, Greaves MW. Cold urticaria treated by induction of tolerance. Lancet. 1979;2:964.
38. Mcdonald SK, Thai KE. Danazol in the treatment of refractory acquired cold urticaria. Australas J Dermatol. 2014;55:303-4.
39. Maurer M, Altrichter S, Metz M, et al. Benefit from reslizumab treatment in a patient with chronic spontaneous urticaria and cold urticaria. J Eur Acad Dermatology Venereol. 2018;32:e112-3.
40. Alangari AA, Twarog FJ, Shih MC, et al. Clinical features and anaphylaxis in children with cold urticaria. Pediatrics. 2004;113:e313-7.
41. Pezzolo E, Peroni A, Gisondi P, et al. Heat urticaria: A revision of published cases with an update on classification and management. Br J Dermatol. 2016;175:473-8.
42. Carballada F, Nuñez R, Martin-Lazaro J, et al. Omalizumab treatment in 2 cases of refractory heat urticaria. J Investig Allergol Clin Immunol. 2013;23:519-21.
43. Quintero OP, Arrondo AP, Veleiro B. Rapid response to omalizumab in 3 cases of delayed pressure urticaria. J Allergy Clin Immunol Pract. 2017;5:179-80.
44. Curto-Barredo L, Archilla LR, Vives GR, et al. Clinical features of chronic spontaneous urticaria that predict disease prognosis and refractoriness to standard treatment. Acta Derm Venereol. 2018;98:641-7.
45. Barlow RJ, Warburton F, Watson K, et al. Diagnosis and incidence of delayed pressure urticaria in patients with chronic urticaria. J Am Acad Dermatol. 1993;29:954-8.
46. Morioke S, Takahagi S, Iwamoto K, et al. Pressure challenge test and histopathological inspections for 17 Japanese cases with clinically diagnosed delayed pressure urticaria. Arch Dermatol Res. 2010;302:613-7.
47. Grundmann SA, Kiefer S, Luger TA, et al. Delayed pressure urticaria—dapsone heading for first-line therapy? J Dtsch Dermatol Ges. 2011;9:908-12.
48. Swerlick RA, Puar N. Delayed pressure urticaria: Response to treatment with sulfasalazine in a case series of seventeen patients. Dermatol Ther. 2015;28:318-22.
49. Eskeland S, Tanum L, Halvorsen JA. Delayed pressure urticaria treated with the selective serotonin reuptake inhibitor escitalopram. Clin Exp Dermatol. 2016;41:526-8.

50. Lawlor F, Black AK, Ward AM, et al. Delayed pressure urticaria, objective evaluation of a variable disease using a dermographometer and assessment of treatment using colchicine. Br J Dermatol. 1989;120:403-8.
51. Pérez-Ferriols A, Barnadas M, Gardeazábal J, et al. Solar urticaria: Epidemiology and clinical phenotypes in a Spanish series of 224 patients. Actas Dermosifiliogr. 2017;108:132-9.
52. Haylett AK, Koumaki D, Rhodes LE. Solar urticaria in 145 patients: Assessment of action spectra and impact on quality of life in adults and children. Photodermatol Photoimmunol Photomed. 2018;doi: 10.1111/phpp.12385. [Epub ahead of print].
53. Morgado-Carrasco D, Fustà-Novell X, Podlipnik S, et al. Clinical and photobiological response in eight patients with solar urticaria under treatment with omalizumab, and review of the literature. Photodermatol Photoimmunol Photomed. 2018;34:194-9.
54. Aubin F, Avenel-Audran M, Jeanmougin M, et al. Omalizumab in patients with severe and refractory solar urticaria: A phase II multicentric study. J Am Acad Dermatol. 2016;74:574-5.
55. Abajian M, Schoepke N, Altrichter S, et al. Physical urticarias and cholinergic urticaria. Immunol Allergy Clin North Am. 2014;34:73-88.
56. Keahey TM, Indrisano J, Lavker RM, et al. Delayed vibratory angioedema: Insights into pathophysiologic mechanisms. J Allergy Clin Immunol. 1987;80:831-8.
57. Metzger WJ, Kaplan AP, Beaven MA, et al. Hereditary vibratory angioedema: Confirmation of histamine release in a type of physical hypersensitivity. J Allergy Clin Immunol. 1976;57:605-8.
58. Boyden SE, Desai A, Cruse G, et al. Vibratory urticaria associated with a missense variant in ADGRE2. N Engl J Med. 2016;374:656-63.
59. Pressler A, Grosber M, Halle M, et al. Failure of omalizumab and successful control with ketotifen in a patient with vibratory angio-oedema. Clin Exp Dermatol. 2013;38:151-3.
60. Ruft J, Asady A, Staubach P, et al. Development and validation of the Cholinergic Urticaria Quality-of-Life Questionnaire (CholU-QoL). Clin Exp Allergy. 2018;48:433-44.
61. Kim JE, Jung KH, Cho HH, et al. The significance of hypersensitivity to autologous sweat and serum in cholinergic urticaria: Cholinergic urticaria may have different subtypes. Int J Dermatol. 2015;54:771-7.
62. Washio K, Fukunaga A, Onodera M, et al. Clinical characteristics in cholinergic urticaria with palpebral angioedema: Report of 15 cases. J Dermatol Sci. 2017;85:135-7.
63. Asady A, Ruft J, Ellrich A, et al. Cholinergic urticaria patients of different age groups have distinct features. Clin Exp Allergy. 2017;47:1609-14.
64. Altrichter S, Koch K, Church MK, et al. Atopic predisposition in cholinergic urticaria patients and its implications. J Eur Acad Dermatology Venereol. 2016;30:2060-5.
65. Vadas P, Sinilaite A, Chaim M. Cholinergic urticaria with anaphylaxis: An underrecognized clinical entity. J Allergy Clin Immunol Pract. 2016;4:284-91.
66. Altrichter S, Salow J, Ardelean E, et al. Development of a standardized pulse-controlled ergometry test for diagnosing and investigating cholinergic urticaria. J Dermatol Sci. 2014;75:88-93.
67. Rothbaum R, McGee JS. Aquagenic urticaria: Diagnostic and management challenges. J Asthma Allergy. 2016;9:209-13.
68. Treudler R, Tebbe B, Steinhoff M, et al. Familial aquagenic urticaria associated with familial lactose intolerance. J Am Acad Dermatol. 2002;47:611-3.
69. Lelonek E, Matusiak L, Wróbel T, et al. Aquagenic pruritus in polycythemia vera: Clinical characteristics. Acta Derm Venereol. 2018;98:496-500.
70. McGee JS, Kirkorian AY, Pappert AS, et al. An adolescent boy with urticaria to water: Review of current treatments for aquagenic urticaria. Pediatr Dermatol. 2014;31:116-7.

CHAPTER

5

Angioedema

Clive EH Grattan

DEFINITION AND DESCRIPTION

Angioedema is a descriptive term for short-lived reversible deep swellings of the skin, submucosa or both due to transient leakage of plasma from small blood vessels. It may also be used as a disease term to describe an illness characterized by recurrent deep swellings *without* wheals.

Unlike wheals, angioedema swellings do not become red or develop a surrounding flare. They are often painful or uncomfortable rather than itchy. They typically resolve completely within hours or days without bruising or scaling. Angioedema often occurs inside or around the mouth (Fig. 5.1), eyelids or genitalia but may happen anywhere on the body surface. In special circumstances, including hereditary angioedema (HAE), it may also affect the bowel and sometimes the bladder. Angioedema may occur with wheals in up to 50% of patients with urticaria and may also be a feature of anaphylaxis.

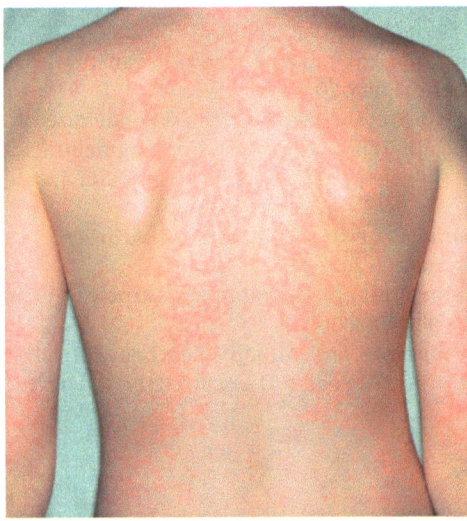

Fig. 5.1: Reticulate erythema preceding an attack of hereditary angioedema.

EPIDEMIOLOGY

Angioedema affects all races, ethnicities, and both sexes equally. The prevalence of HAE is approximately 1:50,000 of the general population (0.00002%). By comparison, the lifetime prevalence of spontaneous urticaria (presenting with wheals, angioedema or both) is said to be 20%. As around 10% of these cases present as angioedema without wheals, it is clear that spontaneous angioedema is very considerably more common than HAE.

CLASSIFICATION

It is helpful from a clinical perspective to separate patients presenting *with* wheals from those *without* wheals since this should determine the initial approach to investigation and management.

- *Angioedema with wheals*: Spontaneous wheals are due to mast cell degranulation with histamine release and secondary mediator generation. In the same way, angioedema in a patient with wheals should be regarded as a manifestation of mast cell dependent urticaria and the stimulus for degranulation should be sought.
- *Angioedema without wheals*: Most cases of angioedema without wheals will be a manifestation of mast cell-dependent acute or chronic spontaneous urticaria (CSU). A very small minority will have an inducible urticaria, including vibratory angioedema. However, of great importance, a few will have acquired or hereditary C1 esterase inhibitor deficiency (HAE with C1-INH deficiency), HAE with normal C1-INH or angiotensin converting enzyme (ACE) inhibitor-induced angioedema due to kinin generation rather than mast cell-derived mediators. Correct identification of kinin-mediated (mast cell-independent) angioedema is essential for appropriate assessment and management, which is completely different from the management of mast cell-dependent angioedema.

PATHOGENESIS

As a working generalization, angioedema is either mast cell-dependent or mast cell-independent, although making this distinction in the clinic may not be easy. The terms histaminergic and nonhistaminergic angioedema are also used. The recognizable etiologies of both groups are summarized in Box 5.1.

Mast Cell-dependent Angioedema

Possible etiologies of spontaneous angioedema include type I allergy to exogenous allergens (acute disease), functional autoantibodies against immunoglobulin E (IgE) or the high affinity IgE receptor (FcεRI), pseudoallergy to nonsteroidal anti-inflammatory drugs (NSAIDs) or food, chronic infection and 'idiopathic' disease (when no single cause can be identified). A concept of type I autoallergy to endogenous allergens as a cause of CSU is emerging. In practice, the majority of patients will have idiopathic angioedema after potential causes have been looked for and excluded as far as possible. Whether a specific cause can be identified or not, it should be recognized that there are multiple potential aggravating factors that worsen but do not cause the illness and these should be revealed by careful history-taking. They include acute

> **Box 5.1:** Etiology of angioedema.
>
> *Mast cell-dependent angioedema:*
> - Spontaneous urticaria (angioedema with wheals and histaminergic angioedema without wheals)
>   – *Acute:*
>   - Idiopathic (the majority)
>   - Post-viral (mainly upper respiratory tract infections)
>   - Allergic (IgE-mediated)
>   - NSAID-induced
>   – *Chronic:*
>   - Idiopathic
>   - Autoimmune (secondary to functional autoantibodies)
>   - Autoallergic
>   - Pseudoallergic (dietary intolerance)
> - *Inducible urticarias:*
>   – Vibratory angioedema
>   – Cholinergic urticaria (may rarely present with angioedema alone)
>
> *Mast cell-independent angioedema:*
> - Acquired C1 esterase inhibitor deficiency
>   – Type 1 (associated with B-cell lymphoproliferative disease, including myeloma)
>   – Type 2 (associated with autoantibodies against C1-INH)
>   – Angiotensin converting enzyme inhibitor-induced
>
> *Hereditary angioedema:*
> - Type I (reduced C1-INH levels and function)
> - Type II (reduced C1-INH function but normal levels)
> - HAE with normal C1-INH
>
> (HAE: hereditary angioedema; IgE: immunoglobulin E; NSAID: nonsteroidal anti-inflammatory drug; C1-INH: C1 esterase inhibitor)

viral upper respiratory tract infections, food intolerance, local heat and pressure and, possibly, stress. Patients presenting with spontaneous angioedema without wheals that responds to antihistamines can be assumed to have mast cell-dependent angioedema.

Mast Cell-independent Angioedema

These patients present *without* wheals and are therefore easily distinguished from the majority of angioedema patients who present *with* wheals. Some families with HAE develop a characteristic prodromal reticulate pattern of erythema (but not whealing, Fig. 5.2) that has been likened to erythema marginatum (first described with rheumatic fever). Mast cell-independent angioedema has a number of causes. Bradykinin appears to be the primary mediator. Acute attacks can be successfully treated with the bradykinin B2 receptor antagonist, icatibant.

- Reduced C1 esterase inhibitor (C1-INH) function may be genetic or acquired. Hereditary C1-INH deficiency is due to mutations in the *SERPING 1* gene on chromosome 1q. Hereditary angioedema may be type I (reduced C1-INH production, seen in 85%) or type II (normal C1-INH levels but reduced C1-INH function, seen in 15%). Acquired angioedema (AAE) is very rare. It is either due to excessive consumption of C1-INH from sustained activation of the classical complement pathway by monoclonal antibodies resulting from B-cell malignancies (type 1 AAE) or production of autoantibodies against C1-INH itself resulting in ineffective binding of the inhibitor to C1. This in turn leads to excessive consumption of C1-INH (type 2 AAE). The regulatory role of C1-INH in the contact, coagulation, fibrinolysis, and complement pathways is shown in Flowchart 5.1.

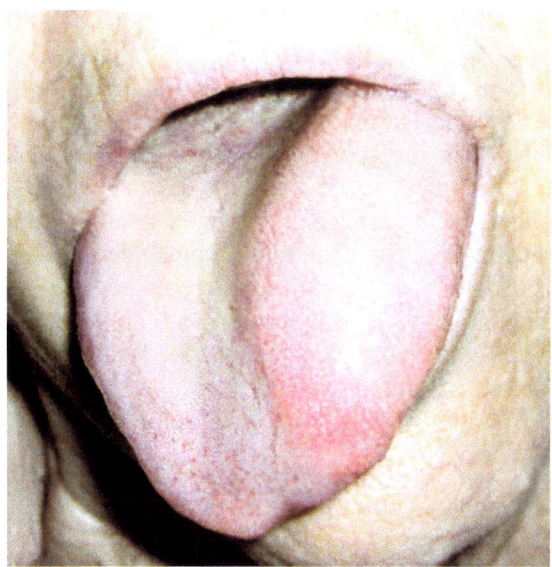

Fig. 5.2: Angioedema affecting one side of the tongue.

Flowchart 5.1: The regulatory function of C1-INH in the contact, clotting, fibrinolysis, and complement systems.

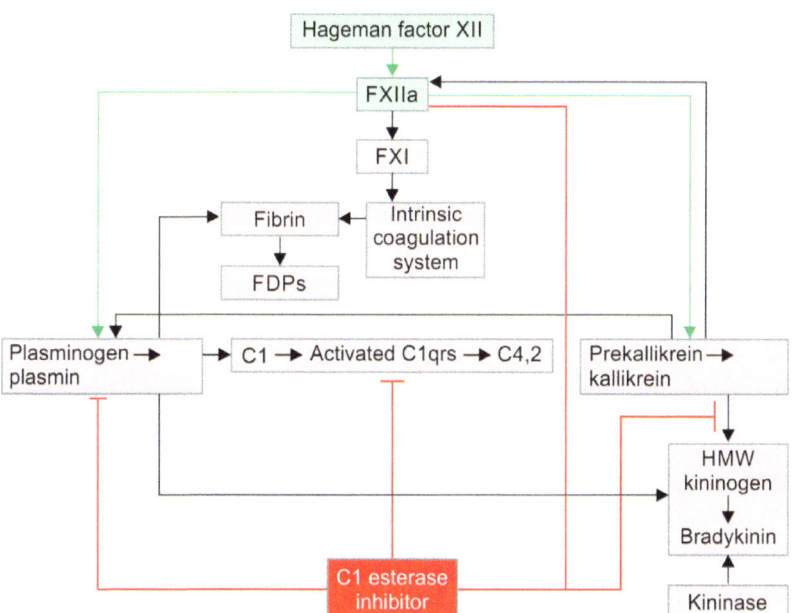

(FDPs: fibrin degradation products; HMW: high-molecular-weight)
Note: The diagram illustrates the key role of C1 esterase inhibitor in controlling not only the complement and coagulation pathways but also the kallikrein-kinin pathways. It is excessive activation of this that leads to hereditary angioedema. The mast cell is not involved.

- Some patients with nonhistaminergic angioedema have normal C1-INH during and between attacks of angioedema. The term HAE with normal C1-INH has been introduced for patients presenting with recurrent angioedema and a positive family history of angioedema without wheals who behave as if they have classical HAE but, nevertheless, have normal C1-INH function and no mutation in *SERPING 1*. About 20% of these patients have been shown to have a mutation of *F12* resulting in autoactivation of Factor XII to FXIIa, especially under the influence of endogenous or exogenous estrogen, resulting in increased activation of the kallikrein-kinin pathway. Novel mutations in angiopoietin 1 gene (*ANGPT1*) and the plasminogen gene (*PLG*) have also been described recently.[1]
- The other important group of patients presenting with nonhistaminergic angioedema are those on ACE inhibitors (ACEi). It is thought that kinin levels increase because bradykinin metabolism by kininase 2 is inhibited by ACEi.

CLINICAL PRESENTATION

Patients presenting with spontaneous mast cell-dependent angioedema usually develop itchy wheals as well, which are often the predominant feature of the illness whatever its etiology. Spontaneous angioedema without wheals is uncommon by comparison. Most cases of this are idiopathic (no definable etiology).

By comparison, patients presenting with mast cell-independent angioedema have deep swellings without wheals that do not itch. The swellings in HAE types I and II are episodic rather than continuous. There are often long intervals between attacks but they may be frequent in some individuals at certain times, for instance during stress, trauma, intercurrent infection or in affected women on estrogen therapy. Not all patients will have a positive family history. About 25% of mutations are sporadic. The angioedema is non-pitting. It may affect the extremities, face, oropharynx, gastrointestinal or genitourinary tracts. The attacks tend to worsen over 24 hours and then take 2–3 days to subside without treatment. About 50% of the attacks affect the gastrointestinal tract and this will present with abdominal colic with vomiting if obstruction of the bowel is complete. It is common for patients to present initially as an acute surgical abdomen and may have unnecessary surgery. Up to 50% of patients experience at least one swelling of the oropharynx over their lifetime, with a real danger of suffocation. Although the diagnosis of HAE is not usually made in new kindreds or sporadic mutations before the second or third decade of life, about 50% of patients have their first attack by the age of 10 years and 75% by 15 years of age. It is uncommon for affected children to develop swellings when less than 6 years old even though diagnostic blood abnormalities may be present from the age of 1 year onward. The influence of pregnancy is variable. The presentation of patients with HAE with normal C1-INH is similar but here a family history if essential for diagnosis, the swellings are less likely to present prior to puberty, there are fewer abdominal attacks and attack-free intervals are often longer.

Acquired angioedema presents in an older population without a family history but the clinical features are otherwise similar to HAE. ACEi-associated angioedema occurs in about 1% of patients prescribed ACEi with a higher proportion in Afro-Caribbean Americans. Swellings usually affect the lower face, lips, and tongue. The interval between starting an ACEi and developing a first attack of angioedema may be as short as a week but a minority of patients present months or even years after commencing therapy so a connection with the medication may not be obvious.

INVESTIGATION

The differential diagnosis of angioedema with respective laboratory profiles is shown in Flowchart 5.2. Patients with wheals should be investigated for underlying causes or associations with spontaneous urticaria. These may include a full blood count, erythrocyte sedimentation rate (ESR), thyroid antibodies and thyroid function as a baseline. Patients presenting with angioedema without wheals, on the other hand, need C4 complement as an initial blood investigation.[2] Normal C4 *during* an attack of angioedema excludes C1-INH deficiency but normal C4 *between* attacks may be found in a few patients with HAE, especially in those on treatment with anabolic steroids. In general, C4 is a quick, inexpensive and sensitive screening test for C1-INH deficiency but is normal in type III HAE. Low C4 is, however, not specific for HAE since reduced levels may also be due to complement consumption in hypocomplementemic urticarial vasculitis or in patients with a C4 null gene. As a guide, C4 levels should be less than 30% of the mean normal laboratory range to be (almost) diagnostic of types I or II HAE.

Patients with low C4 and those with a highly suspicious story of C1-INH deficiency should have quantitative and functional studies of C1-INH to confirm or refute the diagnosis and to distinguish between types I and II HAE. Type I HAE is characterized by reduced levels of C1-INH due to reduced production as a result of a mutation in *SERPING 1*. Around 85% of HAE with C1-INH deficiency have this type. Patients with HAE with normal C1-INH have normal or slightly increased levels of C1-INH but it is nonfunctional due to other mutations in *SERPING 1*. Mutational analysis of *SERPING 1* is only rarely performed in clinical practice because the immunological and biochemical changes in HAE types I and II are nearly always diagnostic.

By contrast, the investigation of HAE with normal C1-INH shows normal C4 and C1-INH function. The pathogenesis of angioedema in patients without a mutation in *F12, ANGPT1* or *PDG* is unknown.

Flowchart 5.2: Differential diagnosis of angioedema and summary of diagnostic investigations.

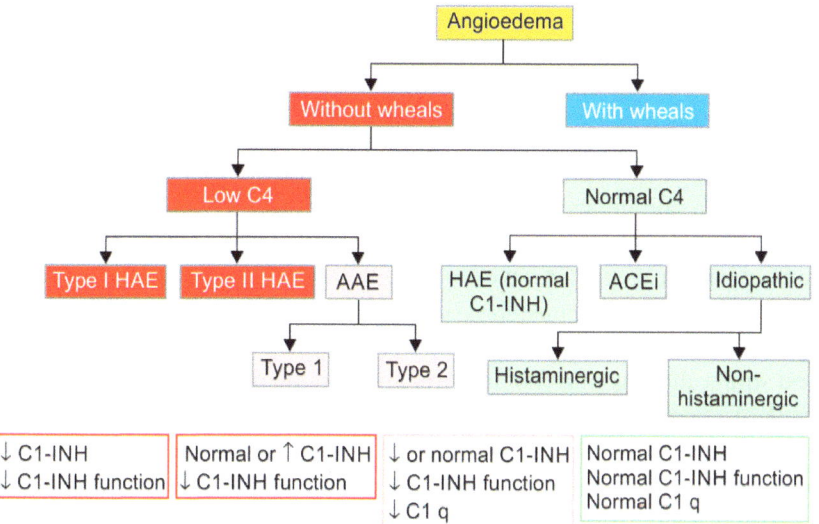

(HAE: hereditary angioedema; AAE: acquired angioedema; ACEi: angiotensin converting enzyme inhibitors)

Patients with AAE have reduced levels of C4, C1-INH and low C1-INH function. Patients with both types 1 and 2 will have low levels of C1q and this can be used as a guide to distinguish AAE from type I HAE.

The role of food additives in precipitating or aggravating idiopathic angioedema may be investigated with single-blind challenges in centers where these are available. Suspected food allergies should be investigated with ImmunoCAP® assay or skin prick testing for specific IgE, when indicated by the history.

MANAGEMENT

Mast Cell-dependent Angioedema

Patients with mast cell-dependent angioedema should be managed in the same way as spontaneous urticaria. In brief, acute or recurrent episodes should be treated with a nonsedating H1 antihistamine with or without short courses of oral corticosteroids (e.g. 0.5 mg/kg/day or equivalent) until the condition has stabilized. Intramuscular epinephrine may also be given for acute oropharyngeal edema if there is a risk of upper airway compromise. A stepwise approach should be adopted for angioedema seen in CSU, starting with the licensed dose of a nonsedating H1 antihistamine, followed by a trial of updosing to fourfold in nonresponders. Some patients will benefit from the addition of targeted but unlicensed "second-line" therapies, including montelukast, and tranexamic acid. Tranexamic acid may be particularly helpful for some patients with idiopathic angioedema without wheals as well as HAE. Omalizumab (anti-IgE) for antihistamine-unresponsive CSU is now recommended as third-line treatment (including patients with predominant angioedema) after updosing of H1 antihistamines, on the basis of good evidence for its use and low side effect profile.[2] "Third-line" immunosuppressive therapies are often used for patients with severe unresponsive CSU but are more likely to be successful in those with evidence of functional autoantibodies (positive autoreactivity on the autologous serum skin test, positive histamine release on the basophil histamine release assay or both) than those without.

Mast Cell-independent Angioedema

Angioedema due to kinin generation or reduced metabolism should be managed completely differently from mast cell-dependent angioedema. Antihistamines are ineffective. Steroids and epinephrine are said not to work although they are often administered for ACEi-induced angioedema in the emergency room. Controlled comparisons against observation alone or active treatment with epinephrine have not been undertaken.

The management of HAE is considered separately for the acute emergency situation, short-term prophylaxis and long-term maintenance (Table 5.1). The principles are the same for children and adults although the choice of treatment in the pediatric population[3] is somewhat limited by risk of adverse effects and licensing restrictions.

- *Acute emergencies*: Intravenous administration of purified C1-INH is a gold standard treatment for facial, oropharyngeal and gastrointestinal swellings causing abdominal colic in children and adults. Consensus opinion based on widespread clinical experience suggests that 500-1,500 U of C1-INH is effective treatment[4] but a recent controlled study in HAE

Table 5.1: Treatment of kinin-mediated angioedema.

	Adults	Children (0–16 years)
	(Optimal dose, usual range)	
Acute emergency situation (central or abdominal swellings)		
pd-C1-INH (IV)	20 U/kg (500–1,500 U)	20 U/kg (500–1,500 U)
Icatibant (S/C)	30 mg (30–90 mg in 24 h)	Weight adjusted (10–30 mg)
Ecallantide (S/C)	30 mg (30–60 mg in 24 h)	
rh-C1-INH (IV)	50 U/kg (4,200 U if ≥ 84 kg, 50–100 U/kg if < 84 kg in 24 h)	
If no pd-C1-INH available, consider: Fresh frozen plasma	10 mL/kg (2–4 U)	10 mL/kg (1–2 U)
Short-term prophylaxis		
pd-C1-INH (IV) 1–24 h before procedure	1,000 U (500–1,500 U)	500 U (500–1,000 U)
Tranexamic acid (po) 2/7 before and after procedure	1g qds	500 mg qds
Danazol (po) 5/7 before and 2/7 after procedure	600 mg (400–600 mg)	300 (2.5–10 mg/kg/day)
Stanozolol (po) 5/7 before and 2/7 after procedure, not usually recommended in children	6 mg (4–6 mg)	
Long-term maintenance		
Tranexamic acid (po)	20–50 mg/kg (1–4.5 g daily)	20–50 mg/kg (1.0–2.0 g daily)
ε-amino caproic acid (po)	3 g (2–6.0)	0.025–0.1 g/kg
Danazol (po)	100 mg (100 mg every 3/7–200 mg daily)	
Rarely used in young children		
Stanozolol (po)	2 mg (2 mg every 3/7–5 mg daily)	
Rarely used in young children		
pd-C1-INH (IV) Pregnancy or intolerance of other prophylactic medications	1000 U × 2/week	

(pd-C1-INH: plasma-derived C1 esterase inhibitor; S/C: subcutaneous; rh-C1-INHL recombinant human C1-INH)

patients at least 6 years old showed that 20 U/kg provided a significant reduction in time to onset of relief compared to placebo but not 10 U/kg.[5] The earliest improvement in symptoms is seen within 40–60 minutes. Complete resolution of the acute attack occurs within less than 12 hours. Single peripheral swellings (not involving the face) may be treated with analgesia alone. Nanofiltered purified C1-INHibitor (nf-C1-INH), recombinant human C1-INH (rh-C1-INH)[6] and a kallikrein inhibitor (ecallantide)[7] are now also available. Of special note, the half-life of rh-C1-INH is shorter than plasma-derived C1 esterase inhibitor (pd-C1-INH) (4 h vs 48 h) and the product is developed from rabbit's milk so patients allergic to rabbits should not be treated with it. A low risk of anaphylaxis after administration of ecallantide presents a small additional hazard to patients who require emergency treatment anyway for their angioedema. Slow, deep subcutaneous injection of 30 mg icatibant,[8] achieves comparable clinical outcomes to pd-C1-INH therapy. Icatibant is the treatment of choice for some patients, especially those suitable for home therapy administered by healthcare professionals or self-administered by the patient. Fresh frozen plasma (10 mL/kg, 2–4 units), containing C1-INH, has been used historically in an emergency as an alternative to pd-C1-INH but has the disadvantage of not being subject to the same rigorous screening for transmissible infection applied to commercial C1-INH products and contains complement, the substrate for C1-INH. Patency of the airway is the top priority in HAE affecting the oropharynx. Tracheostomy may be necessary. Analgesia should be given and intravenous fluids may be required. Recognition of abdominal swelling due to C1-INH deficiency will avoid unnecessary surgery. H1 antihistamines are ineffective since histamine is not a mediator of the swellings.

- *Short-term prophylaxis*: C1-INH should be given to patients with types I or II HAE or AAE 1 hour before major surgery, especially involving intubation. The usual dose is 500–1,000 units with an option of an additional dose afterward if swellings develop. Prophylactic C1-INH may also be considered for dental work involving local anesthesia. For patients already on tranexamic acid or anabolic steroids, the dose can be increased in line with recommended guidelines 5 days before and 2 days after surgery.[4]
- *Long-term prophylaxis*: The disease activity of C1-INH varies over a patient's lifetime and the need for prophylactic treatment will also vary. A few patients with proven HAE will remain attack-free throughout their lives and do not need treatment. At the other end of the spectrum, patients may have multiple peripheral, central or abdominal attacks several times a week and require long-term prophylaxis. A concentrated formulation of C1-INH has been developed for subcutaneous administration.[9] A novel kallikrein inhibitor, lanadelumab, has also been trialled successfully.[10] There is no single approach that suits all individuals and breakthrough attacks should be treated as described above. Patients should try to identify and avoid situations that may trigger angioedema, including ACEi, estrogen therapy, intercurrent infections, *Helicobacter pylori* gastritis, stress and tiredness. The management of kinin-dependent angioedema in children and pregnant women deserves special consideration.
  - *Nonpregnant adults*: Anabolic steroids can be effective but should be monitored with tests of liver function and blood lipids. Three-yearly ultrasound examinations of the liver should also be performed to screen for development of hepatic adenoma. The lowest dose that controls symptoms should be used without reference to quantitative or functional C1-INH levels. Virilizing side effects, including hirsutism, acne, and oligomenorrhea may be unacceptable to women. Danazol and stanozolol are most commonly used but are not available in all countries. Danazol is used at between 100–400 mg daily with some patients being controlled with as little as 100 mg, 5 days a week. Stanozolol is used at 2–6 mg daily but some patients may manage on as little as 2 mg three times a week. Tranexamic acid is a plasmin inhibitor. It is taken at doses ranging from 20 mg/kg to 40 mg/kg. Changes in color vision, as evidence of retinal microvascular thrombosis, need to be reported by patients promptly. Those with a personal or strong family history of thrombosis should not be treated. Liver function tests should be monitored at least once every 3 months initially. Tranexamic acid is more likely to be useful in HAE with normal C1-INH than danazol (or equivalent) but danazol is more likely to be effective than tranexamic acid in HAE types I and II.

- *Pregnant or lactating women*: Tranexamic acid can be taken throughout pregnancy and breast-feeding provided it is effective. Anabolic steroids are contraindicated should be avoided. A few women require twice weekly infusions of C1-INH as prophylaxis throughout their pregnancy and sometimes beyond. Icatibant is currently not recommended for pregnant or lactating women.
- *Childhood*: Since up to 75% of children develop an attack of angioedema before their 15th birthday, about half will require long-term or intermittent prophylaxis. Tranexamic acid is more appropriate than anabolic steroids, which carry a risk of growth retardation due to premature closure of the epiphyses.

SUMMARY

Patients presenting with angioedema without wheals are a small but important subgroup of patients presenting with angioedema. The majority of patients with angioedema without wheals will have histaminergic mast cell-dependent disease. A minority will have kinin-mediated mast cell-independent angioedema that may or may not be due to C1-INH deficiency or dysfunction. For these, there has been a recent investment by the pharmaceutical industry resulting in the development of important novel therapies that block key steps in the contact (kallikrein-kinin) pathway in addition to the replacement of missing or defective C1-INH that remains the gold standard management of acute severe attacks for now.

REFERENCES

1. Zuraw BL. Hereditary angioedema with normal C1-INHibitor: Four types and counting. J Allergy Clin Immunol. 2018;141:884-5.
2. Zuberbier T, Aberer W, Asero R, et al. The EAACI/GA²LEN/EDF/WAO guideline for the definition, classification, diagnosis and management of urticaria. Allergy. 2018;73:1393-414.
3. Ebo DG, Vermeil MM, de Knop KJ, et al. Hereditary angioedema in childhood. An approach to management. Pediatric Drugs. 2010;12:257-68.
4. Gompels MM, Lock RJ, Abinun M, et al. C1-INHibitor deficiency: Consensus document. Clin Exp Immunol. 2005;139:379-94.
5. Craig TJ, Levy RJ, Wasserman RL, et al. Efficacy of human C1 esterase inhibitor concentrate compared with placebo in acute hereditary angioedema. J Allergy Clin Immunol. 2009;124:801-8.
6. Zuraw B, Cicardi M, Levy RJ, et al. Recombinant human C1-inhibitor for the treatment of acute angioedema attacks in patients with hereditary angioedema. J Allergy Clin Immunol. 2010;126:821-7.
7. Sheffer AL, Campion M, Levy RJ, et al. Ecallantide (DX-88) for acute hereditary angioedema attacks: Integrated analysis of 2 double-blind, phase 3 studies. J Allergy Clin Immunol. 2011;128:153-9.
8. Lumry WR, Li HH, Levy RJ, et al. Randomized placebo-controlled trial of the bradykinin B(2) receptor antagonist icatibant for the treatment of acute attacks of hereditary angioedema: the FAST-3 trial. Ann Allergy Asthma Immunol. 2011;107:529-37.
9. Longhurst H, Cicardi M, Craig T, et al. Prevention of hereditary angioedema attacks with a subcutaneous C1 inhibitor. N Engl J Med. 2017;376:1131-40.
10. Banerji A, Busse P, Shennak M, et al. Inhibiting plasma kallikrein for hereditary angioedema prophylaxis. N Engl J Med. 2017;376:717-28.

CHAPTER 6

Cutaneous Mastocytosis

Frank Siebenhaar

DEFINITION

Mastocytosis is a heterogeneous disease belonging to the group myeloproliferative disorders characterized by pathological increase and accumulation of mast cells in the skin (cutaneous mastocytosis) and/or internal organs, such as bone marrow, liver, spleen, and the lymph nodes (systemic mastocytosis).

CLASSIFICATION

By definition, cutaneous mastocytosis only affects the skin and is the most common form of mastocytosis, mainly present in children. Most adult patients present with indolent systemic mastocytosis, in about 85% with mastocytosis in the skin (Flowchart 6.1).

Flowchart 6.1: Classification of mastocytosis.

```
                              Mastocytosis
                                   │
        ┌──────────────────────────┼──────────────────────────┐
        ▼                          ▼                          ▼
Cutaneous mastocytosis    Mastocytosis in the         Systemic mastocytosis
       (CM)                   skin (MIS)                      (SM)
(Systemic involvement    (Systemic involvement         (Confirmed by WHO
    excluded)                  unknown)                      criteria)
```

- Cutaneous mastocytosis (CM) branches into: Maculopapular CM (Syn. urticaria pigmentosa), Diffuse CM (Children), Cutaneous mastocytoma (Children)
- Maculopapular CM branches into: Monomorphic (Adults), Monomorphic (Children)
- Systemic mastocytosis (SM):
  - Indolent systemic mastocytosis (ISM)
  - Isolated bone marrow mastocytosis (BMM)
  - Smoldering systemic mastocytosis (SSM)
  - SM with associated hematologic neoplasm (SM-AHN)
  - Aggressive systemic mastocytosis (ASM)
  - Mast cell leukemia
  - Mast cell sarcoma

EPIDEMIOLOGY

Approximate prevalence of mastocytosis is estimated to 2–3/10,000 inhabitants. Thus, mastocytosis belongs to the group of orphan diseases.
- *Age*: About half of the cases occur in early childhood with frequent onset during infancy.
- *Sex*: No predilection.
- *Prevalence*: Worldwide disease.

ETIOLOGY AND PATHOGENESIS

Cutaneous mastocytosis is usually a sporadic disorder. Familial predisposition has been occasionally reported. It is well established that somatic activating mutations in exon 17 of c-kit play a crucial role in the pathogenesis of mastocytosis. The most common is D816V mutation, which affects about 90% of adults. In children, other mutations of c-kit have been described including K839E, D816Y, D816F, D816I, and R815K as well as mutations in exons 8, 9, and 11 of c-kit. Familial cases occasionally present with germline mutations of c-kit.

CLINICAL FEATURES

About 50% of patients of cutaneous mastocytosis present within first few months of life. It is usually an asymptomatic disease; however, parents are concerned about the lesions that appear as multiple pigmented macules on the body. In contrast to adults, who present with typical monomorphic lesions, known as urticaria pigmentosa (Fig. 6.1), children often show larger and polymorphic lesions (Fig. 6.2).

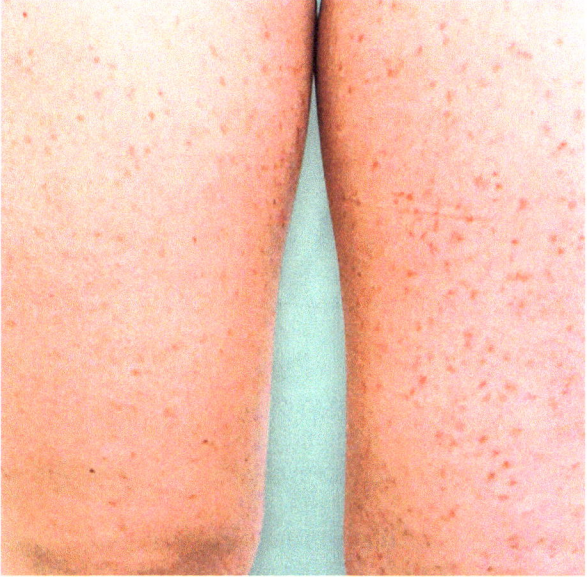

Fig. 6.1: An adult with urticaria pigmentosa (monomorphic).

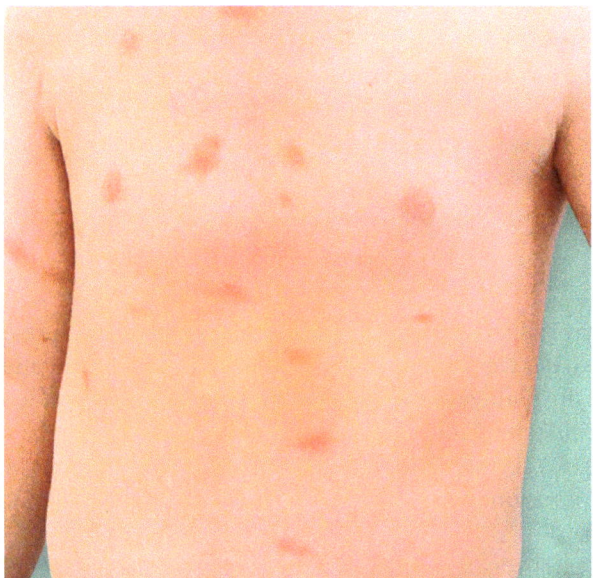

Fig. 6.2: A child with polymorphic pigmented lesions.

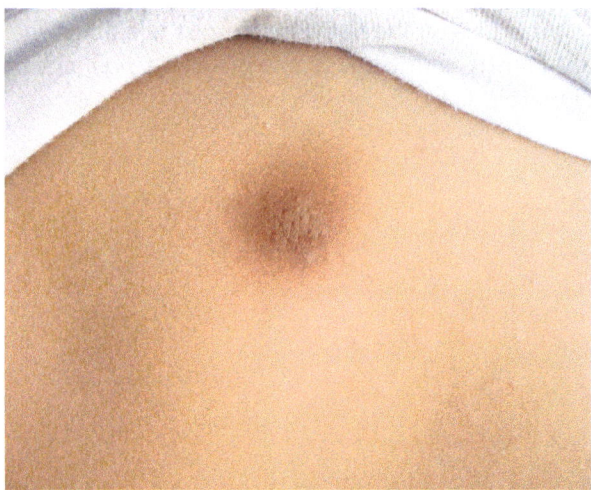

Fig. 6.3: A young adult patient with solitary mastocytoma, demonstrating Darier's sign.

Sudden urtication of skin lesions by gentle stroking, trauma or friction is known as Darier's sign, which is pathognomonic for cutaneous mastocytosis (Fig. 6.3). Thus, palpation or rubbing of the lesions allows for easy diagnosis of cutaneous mastocytosis, which should not be missed. In small children, Darier's sign should be provoked with caution due to the risk of inducing systemic symptoms.

Extensive disease, as in diffuse cutaneous mastocytosis, may present with brown-black nodules and plaques, which virtually affect the entire skin. In infants, bullae may frequently occur at the site of friction or trauma. Rarely, the plaques or nodules may be of yellowish, creamy appearance in a variant called xanthelasmoid mastocytosis. Solitary plaques or nodules are rare. All these lesions are suspected to be part of mastocytosis based on the clinical demonstration of Darier's sign. Infrequently, a telangiectatic variant of maculopapular cutaneous mastocytosis is observed, which mainly presents in adults. Telangiectasia macularis eruptiva perstans (TMEP) has been removed from the current classification, since the term is confusing.

Depending on the extent of the disease, other symptoms resulting from mast cell degranulation, including flushing, diarrhea, vomiting, syncope, or anaphylaxis may occur. Anaphylactic reactions to drugs or hymenoptera stings are common and may be the first sign of mastocytosis.

Systemic mastocytosis exhibit variable clinical features as discussed further in the complications section.

INVESTIGATIONS AND DIAGNOSIS

To confirm the diagnosis a skin biopsy is recommended to demonstrate an increased number of mast cells (Fig. 6.4). However, the histological finding needs to correlate with the clinical picture, since histological criteria for mastocytosis in the skin are missing and various inflammatory skin conditions can give rise to cutaneous mast cell accumulation. Mast cells are not detectable in routine hematoxylin and eosin staining. Therefore, Giemsa or toluidine blue staining is required and helps for easy recognition of the skin mast cells' metachromatic granules (Fig. 6.5).

In bullous mastocytosis, Tzanck smear can demonstrate multiple mast cells may be helpful in making a rapid bedside diagnosis. An important aspect of mast cell disease is early recognition of systemic mastocytosis. The latter should be suspected in all adult patients and exceptionally in children with progressive diffuse cutaneous mastocytosis. In such cases, serum tryptase

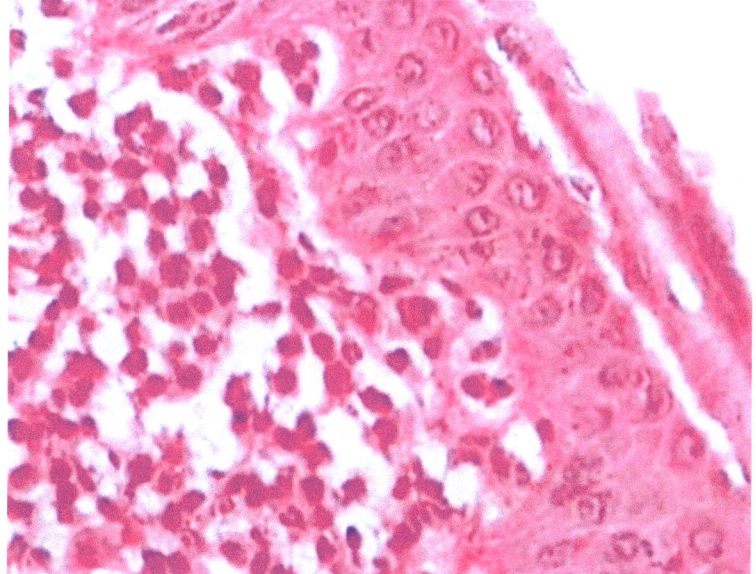

Fig. 6.4: A typical histopathological feature of mastocytosis showing increased numbers of mast cells in the upper dermis.

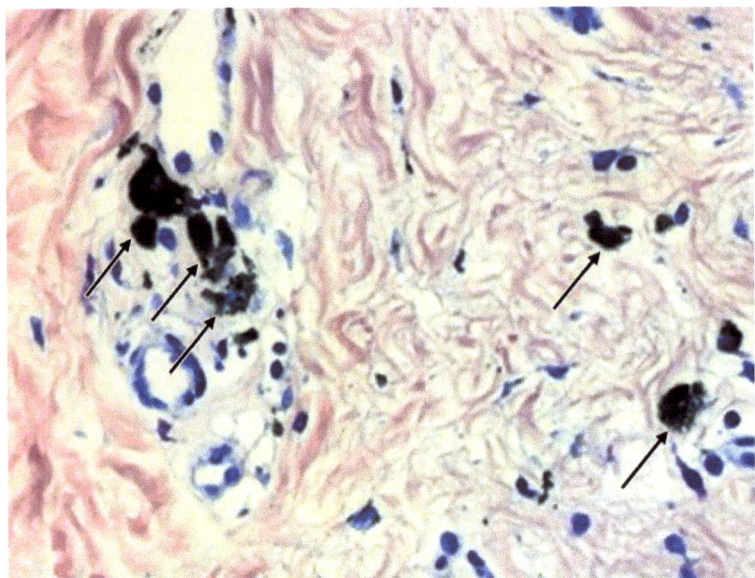

Fig. 6.5: Characteristic metachromatic granules (arrows, Giemsa stain).

levels, bone marrow examination including immunohistochemistry (CD25 on mast cells) and testing for c-kit mutation, as well as radiographs of bones (osteoporosis), and abdominal sonography should be considered. It is recommended to monitor all adult patients for tryptase and differential blood counts at least once a year.

DIFFERENTIAL DIAGNOSIS

Macular lesions may be misdiagnosed in early stage as melanocytic nevi, postinflammatory hyperpigmentation or purpura pigmentosa progressive. Telangiectatic lesions may be confused with idiopathic eruptive macular pigmentation or essential telangiectasia.
- Vesiculobullous lesions of mastocytosis in children may be confused with mastocytosis, staphylococcal scalded skin syndrome, erythema multiforme, and epidermolysis bullosa
- Violaceous plaques of mastocytosis may mimic lichen planus
- Yellow-brown plaques may be misdiagnosed as xanthomas (Fig. 6.6)
- Solitary plaques may be misdiagnosed as fibroma or collagenoma.

SYSTEMIC MASTOCYTOSIS

The WHO criteria for diagnosis of systemic mastocytosis consist of one major and four minor criteria. For the diagnosis of systemic mastocytosis, either the major and one minor criterion or three minor criteria need to be fulfilled.

Major

Multifocal dense infiltrates (>15 mast cells) in bone marrow or other extracutaneous organ.

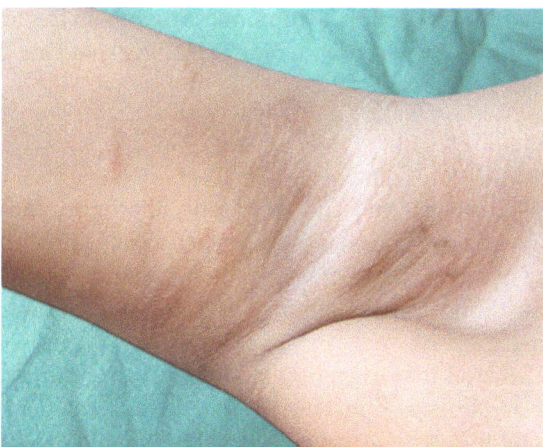

Fig. 6.6: Multiple yellowish creamy plaques along the axilla in a child, mimicking xanthoma.

Minor

- Mast cells in bone marrow or other extracutaneous organ show atypical or spindle-shaped morphology (>25%)
- Codon 816 c-kit mutation in extracutaneous organ
- Mast cells in bone marrow express CD2, CD25, or both
- Basal serum tryptase level constantly greater than 20 ng/mL.

COMPLICATIONS

The range of symptoms depends on the extent of the mast cell disease and the mediators released, as well as the organs involved.

Patients may also have chronic systemic symptoms involving various organ systems, such as the skeletal system (bone pain or pathologic fractures due to osteoporosis), central nervous system (neuropsychiatric symptoms), gastrointestinal involvement (diarrhea, nausea, vomiting, and malabsorption), and cardiovascular symptoms (shock, syncope, and flushing).

General anesthesia is a high-risk procedure, since severe reactions such as systemic hypotension and coagulopathy resulting in death have been reported. A close communication between anesthesiologists, surgeons, and intensive care specialists should be established prior to surgery.

Patients with adult- or adolescent-onset urticaria pigmentosa are more likely to have persistent disease and are at higher risk for systemic involvement. Hence, such patients should be carefully followed up and thoroughly investigated.

TREATMENT

Conservative approach and symptomatic care is all that required for most patients with cutaneous mastocytosis since the prognosis is excellent.

Patients and doctors need to be advised to use drugs that may cause mediator release, such as aspirin and other nonsteroidal anti-inflammatory drugs, codeine, morphine, thiamine, opiates, and contrast media with caution. Symptomatic treatment is mainly based on the use of H_1-antihistamines with or without the combination of H2-blockers. Oral disodium cromoglycate may help gastrointestinal symptoms.

Other Therapy

Leukotriene antagonists, corticosteroids, phototherapy, interferon, and cyclosporine are other therapies reported with variable success. Potent corticosteroids used topically with occlusion may help in controlling pruritus and decreasing the number of lesional mast cells in solitary cutaneous mastocytomas. Short-term systemic steroids may bring dramatic response on diffuse cutaneous or bullous mastocytosis.

Patients should be advised that triggering factors, such as heat, cold, and friction of skin lesions, pressure, exercise, stress, contrast media, and drugs might cause mediator release.

Adult patients and children with history of anaphylaxis should be equipped with emergency medication.

COURSE AND PROGNOSIS

Generally, the prognosis is excellent in childhood-onset mastocytosis with a high rate of remission. Most adult-onset patients suffer from indolent systemic mastocytosis, which is a chronic but stable or very slowly progressing condition. In general, the prognosis is also very good but life quality might be tremendously impaired depending on symptoms. Careful attention should be given to patients with highly elevated tryptase (>200 ng/mL) and/or splenomegaly, since these are signs for an increased risk of progression.

CONCLUSION

Cutaneous mastocytosis is a rare disease and may mimic other dermatological conditions. Childhood mastocytosis is asymptomatic in the majority of the cases and exhibit a high rate of remission. Adult mastocytosis is chronic and frequently includes indolent systemic involvement. Treatment strategies are mainly symptomatic and depend on their intensity. Progression of disease or aggressive forms are rarely seen but should not missed since these conditions usually exhibit reduced life expectancy and need further treatment in collaboration with a hematologist.

BIBLIOGRAPHY

1. Chang A, Tung RC, Schlesinger T, et al. Familial cutaneous mastocytosis. Pediatr Dermatol. 2001;18:271-6.
2. Golitz LE, Weston W, Lane A. Bullous mastocytosis: Diffuse cutaneous mastocytosis with extensive blisters mimicking scalded skin syndrome or erythema multiforme. Pediatr Dermatol. 1984;1:288-94.
3. Hartmann K, Escribano L, Grattan C, et al. Cutaneous manifestations in patients with mastocytosis: Consensus report of the European Competence Network on Mastocytosis; the American Academy of Allergy, Asthma; Immunology; and the European Academy of Allergology and Clinical Immunology. J Allergy Clin Immunol. 2016;137:35-45.
4. Has C, Misery L, David L, et al. Recurring staphylococcal scalded skin syndrome-like bullous mastocytosis: The utility of cytodiagnosis and the rapid regression with steroid. Pediatr Dermatol. 2002;19:220-3.

5. Heide R, Tank B, Orange AP. Mastocytosis in childhood. Pediatr Dermatol. 2002;19:357-81.
6. Husak R, Blume-Peytavi U, Pfrommer C, et al. Nodular and bullous cutaneous mastocytosis of the xanthelasmoid type: Case report. Br J Dermatol. 2001;144:355-8.
7. Inamadar AC, Palit A. Cutaneous mastocytosis: Report of six cases. Indian J Dermatol Venereol Leprol. 2006;72:50-3.
8. Kanwar AJ, Sandhu K. Cutaneous mastocytosis in children: An Indian experience. Pediatr Dermatol. 2005;22:85-7.
9. Lange M, Niedoszytko M, Nedoszytko B, et al. Diffuse cutaneous mastocytosis: Analysis of 10 cases and a brief review of the literature. J Eur Acad Dermatol Venereol. 2012;26:1565-71.
10. Metcalfe DD, Mekori YA. Pathogenesis and pathology of mastocytosis. Annu Rev Pathol. 2017;12:487-514.
11. Siebenhaar F, Akin C, Bindslev-Jensen C, et al. Treatment strategies in mastocytosis. Immunol Allergy Clin North Am. 2014;34:433-47.
12. Valent P, Akin C, Metcalfe DD. Mastocytosis: 2016 updated WHO classification and novel emerging treatment concepts. Blood. 2017;129:1420-7.
13. Vano-Galvan S, De la Hoz B, Nuñez R, et al. Indolent mastocytosis. Isr Med Assoc J. 2010;12:185-7.
14. Verma KK, Bhat R, Singh MK. Bullous mastocytosis treated with oral betamethasone therapy. Indian J Pediatr. 2004;71:261-3.

CHAPTER 7

Pharmacology of Antihistamines

Martin K Church

INTRODUCTION

To understand the strengths and weaknesses of H_1-antihistamines, it is necessary to appreciate how they were developed in the 1930s. In his review about his own work,[1] Daniel Bovet wrote "three naturally occurring amines, acetylcholine, epinephrine, and histamine, may be grouped together because they have a similar chemical structure, are all present in the body fluids, and exert characteristically strong pharmacologic activities. There are alkaloids that interfere with the effects of acetylcholine. Similarly, there are sympatholytic poisons that neutralize or reverse the effects of epinephrine. It seemed possible to me, therefore, that some substance might exist which exerts a specific antagonism toward histamine." It was against this background that Bovet, who was looking for antagonists of acetylcholine, asked his student, Anne-Marie Staub, to test some of these compounds against histamine. This led to the discovery of the first H_1-antihistamine in 1937.[2] Although this compound was too toxic for use in humans, it opened the door for the introduction of the First Generation Antihistamines into the clinic. These included antergan in 1942,[3] followed by diphenhydramine in 1945[4] and chlorpheniramine, brompheniramine, and promethazine later the same decade.[5]

HISTAMINE H_1-RECEPTOR

The histamine H_1-receptor is a member of the superfamily of G-protein coupled receptors (GPCRs). GPCRs, may be viewed as "cellular switches" which exist as an equilibrium between the inactive or "off" state and the active or "on" state.[6] In the case of the histamine H_1-receptor, histamine cross links sites on transmembrane domains III and V to stabilize the receptor in its active conformation thus causing the equilibrium to swing to the "on" position.[7] H_1-antihistamines, which are not structurally related to histamine, do not antagonize the binding of histamine but bind to different sites on the receptor to produce the opposite effect. For example, cetirizine cross links sites on transmembrane domains IV and VI to stabilize the receptor in the inactive state and swing the equilibrium to the "off" position.[8] Thus, H_1-antihistamines are not receptor antagonists but are inverse agonists in that they produce the opposite effect on the receptor to histamine.[6] Consequently, the preferred term to define these drugs is "H_1-antihistamines" rather than "histamine antagonists".

Development of H_1-antihistamines

Bearing in mind that first-generation H_1-antihistamines derive from the same chemical stem from which cholinergic muscarinic antagonists, tranquilizers, antipsychotics, and antihypertensive agents were also developed, it is hardly surprising that they have poor receptor selectivity and often interact with receptors of other biologically active amines causing antimuscarinic, anti-α-adrenergic and anti-serotonin effects.[9] But perhaps their greatest drawback is their ability to cross blood–brain barrier and interfere with histaminergic transmission.

Histamine is an important neuromediator in the human brain which contains approximately 64,000 histamine-producing neurons, emanating from the tuberomammillary nucleus.[10] Stimulation of H_1-receptors in the central nervous system (CNS) increases arousal in the circadian sleep/wake cycle, reinforces learning and memory, and has roles in fluid balance, suppression of feeding, control of body temperature, control of cardiovascular system, and mediation of stress-triggered release of ACTH and β-endorphin from the pituitary gland.[11] It is not surprising then that first-generation H_1-antihistamines, such as chlorpheniramine, diphenhydramine, hydroxyzine and ketotifen, which, even when given at licensed doses, occupy more than 50% of brain H1-receptors interfere with all of these processes (Fig. 7.1).

Physiologically, the release of histamine during the day causes arousal whereas its decreased production at night results in a passive reduction of the arousal response. When taken during the day, first-generation H_1-antihistamines, even in the manufacturers' recommended doses, frequently cause daytime somnolence, sedation, drowsiness, fatigue and impaired concentration and memory.[12,13] When taken at night, first-generation H_1-antihistamines increase the latency to the onset of rapid eye movement (REM) sleep and reduce the duration of REM sleep.[14-16] The

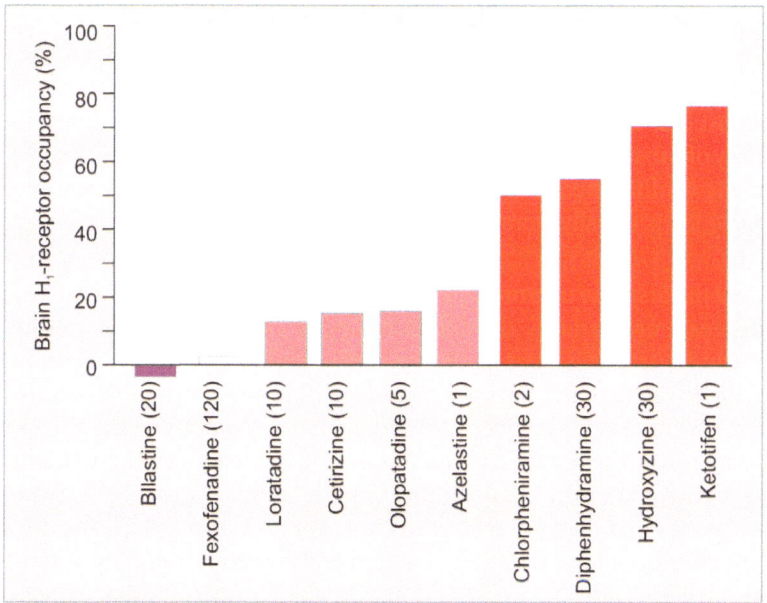

Fig. 7.1: Brain receptor occupancy of H_1-antihistamines.[19,40] The doses of the drugs uses are in parentheses.

residual effects of poor sleep, including impairment of attention, vigilance, working memory and sensory-motor performance, are still present the next morning.[15,17] This is especially problematical with drugs with a long half-life. The detrimental CNS effects of first-generation H_1-antihistamines on learning and examination performance in children and on the impairment of the ability of adults to work, drive and fly aircraft have been reviewed in detail in a recent review.[9]

A major advance in antihistamine development occurred in the 1980s with the introduction of second-generation H_1-antihistamines, including loratadine, desloratadine, cetirizine, levocetirizine, ebastine, azelastine and olopatadine, which have high H_1-receptor selectivity, no anticholinergic effects, low brain permeability, and longer durations of action.[18] Unlike first-generation drugs, second-generation H_1-antihistamines are amphiphilic in that hydrophilic groups have been introduced into the molecule so that they are always positively or negatively charged and, therefore, have a greatly reduced passage across the blood–brain barrier occupying less than 20% of brain H_1-receptors (Fig. 7.1).[19,20] Although second-generation H_1-antihistamines have a much reduced brain penetration, they may only be referred to as "minimally sedating" rather than "non-sedating". For example, in a study of patients' perspective of effectiveness and side effects of H_1-antihistamine updosing in chronic spontaneous urticaria (CSU), more than 20% of patients reported sedation is a side effect of second-generation systemic antihistamines (SGAHs).[21]

More recently, two truly "non-sedating" H_1-antihistamines, fexofenadine, and bilastine, have been introduced which have no significant occupation of histamine H_1-receptors in the central nervous system (Fig. 7.1).[20,22] The reason for their lack of brain penetration is that they are actively pumped out of the blood–brain barrier by p-glycoprotein (a proton pump).[23-25] It will be interesting to see if further drugs will be developed which use membrane proton pumps to enhance their efficacy or reduce their unwanted effects.

H_1-antihistamines in Urticaria

Most types urticaria, including CSU and the majority of inducible urticarias, are mediated primarily by mast cell-derived histamine[26] which reaches very high concentrations due to the poor diffusibility of substances in the dermis.[27,28] Urticaria is characterized by short-lived wheals ranging from a few millimeters to several centimeters in diameter which are accompanied by severe itching which is usually worse in the evening or night-time.[29]

The latest EAACI/GA²LEN/EDF/WAO guidelines for the management of urticaria[30] recommend that the first-line treatment for urticaria should be second-generation, non-sedating H_1-antihistamines. Furthermore, the guidelines state "we recommend aiming at complete symptom control in urticaria, considering as much as possible the safety and the quality of life of each individual patient". Because, standard licensed doses of H_1-antihistamines are often ineffective in completely relieving symptoms in many patients[21] the guidelines state "we suggest updosing second-generation H_1-antihistamines up to four-fold in patients with chronic urticaria unresponsive to second-generation H_1-antihistamines onefold".[30] Thus, it is clear that the attributes that dermatologists seek when choosing an H_1-antihistamine are a rapid onset of action, good efficacy, a long duration of action and freedom from unwanted effects. While some of these attributes may be predicted from preclinical and pharmacokinetic studies, it is only in the clinical environment that they may be definitively established.[31]

Speed of Onset of Action and Duration of Action

The speed of onset of action of a drug is often equated to the rate of its oral absorption and its duration of action by its plasma concentration. However, this is not strictly correct as a time for a drug to diffuse into the extravascular space to produce a maximal clinical effect. In adults, the maximal inhibition of the flare response is usually approximately 4 hours for levocetirizine, fexofenadine, and desloratadine[32-34] but may be longer for drugs, such as loratadine and ebastine, which require metabolism to produce their active moiety.[34]

The duration of action of antihistamines is also much longer than would be predicted from knowledge of their plasma concentration and for most is in the vicinity of 24 hours.[25,35] This is presumably to "trapping" of the drug by its strong and long-lasting binding to histamine H_1-receptors.[8] Because it is actively secreted into the intestine and urine by P-glycoprotein,[23] the duration of action of fexofenadine is shorter, around 8.5 hours[36] indicating that may be best given twice daily. In contrast, bilastine, which is also a substrate for P-glycoprotein, has a duration of action of around 24 hours. The reason for this difference is that bilastine is also a substrate for OATP1A, an intestinal pump that facilitates its uptake into the bloodstream.[25,37] Even so, the guidelines suggest that second-generation H_1-antihistamines should be taken regularly for the treatment of patients with chronic urticaria in order to obtain maximum efficacy.[30]

Efficacy

A question that is asked repeatedly is how the dose of an antihistamine is determined. The answer is that it is a balance between the effectiveness and the unwanted or side effects of a drug. For first-generation H_1-antihistamines, it is the degree somnolence that they cause limits the amount of drug that may be given. Hence, drugs have relative weak efficacy. With most second-generation H_1-antihistamines, their ability to penetrate the CNS sedation is again a limiting factor. Drugs such as cetirizine and desloratadine may be minimally sedating at licensed doses, but updosing may cause sedation in susceptible patients. A possible exception to this rule is bilastine which, because it is a P-glycoprotein substrate and does not penetrate the CNS, is more effective as a single dose and may be updosed without fear of somnolence.[24,25,38]

CLINICAL USAGE

For the treatment of chronic urticaria, the guidelines[30] that treatment should start with a standard single dose second-generation H_1-antihistamine. If adequate control is not achieved after 2–4 weeks, or earlier if symptoms are intolerable, then the dose should be doubled. If adequate control is still not achieved after a further 2–4 weeks, or earlier if symptoms are intolerable, then the dose should be increased to four times the initial dose. The guidelines also recommend updosing with a single antihistamine rather than using different H_1-antihistamines at the same time. If somnolence is a problem then either fexofenadine or bilastine should be considered.

For children, many clinicians use first-generation, sedating H_1-antihistamines as their first choice assuming that the safety profile of these drugs is better known than that of the newer second-generation H_1-antihistamines. However, the guidelines make a strong recommendation to discourage the use of first-generation antihistamines in infants and children for the reasons stated above. Thus, in children the same first-line treatment and updosing (weight and age adjusted) is recommended as in adults. It should be realized, however, that young children have more body water, as a percentage, than adults. Also, their renal function is fully developed. In contrast, liver enzymes mature more slowly reaching maximum at around 10 years of age. Consequently, in young children, only water-soluble drugs that are excreted renally, such as cetirizine, levocetirizine, fexofenadine, and bilastine, should be used.

In elderly patients, again first-generation antihistamines should not be used, particularly those with dementia as cumulative use of first-generation antihistamines with anticholinergic activity is associated with an increased risk for dementia in such patients.[39]

CONCLUSION

In conclusion, the use of first-generation H_1-antihistamines should be discouraged in clinical practice today for two main reasons. First, they are less effective than second-generation H_1-antihistamines.[40] Second, they have unwanted side effects and the potential for causing severe toxic reactions that are not shared by second-generation H_1-antihistamines.

With regard to second-generation H_1-antihistamines, there are many efficacious and safe drugs on the market for the treatment of allergic disease. Of the three drugs highlighted in this review, levocetirizine, fexofenadine, and bilastine are the most potent in humans in vivo. However, levocetirizine may cause somnolence in susceptible individuals while fexofenadine has a relatively short duration of action and may be required to be given twice daily for all round daily protection. While desloratadine is less potent, it has the advantages of rarely causing somnolence and having a long duration of action. Bilastine is perhaps the most effective drug and does not cause somnolence.

REFERENCES

1. Bovet D. Introduction to antihistamine agents and antergan derivative. Ann N Y Acad Sci. 1950;50:1089-126.
2. Staub AM. Action de la thymoxyethyldiethylamine (929F) et des ethers phenoliques sur le choc anaphylactique. Compt Rend Soc Biol. 1937;125:818-21.
3. Halpern BN. Les antihistaminiques de synthese. Essais de chemotherapie des etats allergiques. Arch Int Pharmacodyn Ther. 1942;681:339-408.
4. Loew ER, MacMillan R, Kaiser ME. The anti-histamine properties of benadryl, beta-dimethylaminoethyl benzhydryl ether hydrochloride. J Pharmacol Exp Ther. 1946;86:229-38.
5. Emanuel MB. Histamine and the antiallergic antihistamines: A history of their discoveries. Clin Exp Allergy. 1999;29:1-11.
6. Leurs R, Church MK, Taglialatela M. H1-antihistamines: Inverse agonism, anti-inflammatory actions and cardiac effects. Clin Exp Allergy. 2002;32:489-98.
7. Wieland K, Laak AM, Smit MJ, et al. Mutational analysis of the antagonist-binding site of the histamine H(1) receptor. J Biol Chem. 1999;274:29994-30000.
8. Gillard M, Van Der Perren C, Moguilevsky N, et al. Binding characteristics of cetirizine and levocetirizine to human H(1) histamine receptors: contribution of Lys(191) and Thr(194). Mol Pharmacol. 2002;61:391-9.
9. Church MK, Maurer M, Simons FE, et al. Risk of first-generation H(1)-antihistamines: a GA(2)LEN position paper. Allergy. 2010;65:459-66.
10. Haas H, Panula P. The role of histamine and the tuberomamillary nucleus in the nervous system. Nat Rev Neurosci. 2003;4:121-30.

11. Brown RE, Stevens DR, Haas HL. The physiology of brain histamine. Prog Neurobiol. 2001;63:637-72.
12. Simons FE. Advances in H1-antihistamines. N Engl J Med. 2004;351:2203-17.
13. Juniper EF, Stahl E, Doty RL, et al. Clinical outcomes and adverse effect monitoring in allergic rhinitis. J Allergy Clin Immunol. 2005;115:S390-413.
14. Adam K, Oswald I. The hypnotic effects of an antihistamine: Promethazine. Br J Clin Pharmacol. 1986;22:715-7.
15. Boyle J, Eriksson M, Stanley N, et al. Allergy medication in Japanese volunteers: Treatment effect of single doses on nocturnal sleep architecture and next day residual effects. Curr Med Res Opin. 2006;22:1343-51.
16. Rojas-Zamorano JA, Esqueda-Leon E, Jimenez-Anguiano A, et al. The H1 histamine receptor blocker, chlorpheniramine, completely prevents the increase in REM sleep induced by immobilization stress in rats. Pharmacol Biochem Behav. 2009;91:291-4.
17. Kay GG, Berman B, Mockoviak SH, et al. Initial and steady-state effects of diphenhydramine and loratadine on sedation, cognition, mood, and psychomotor performance. Arch Intern Med. 1997;157:2350-6.
18. Holgate ST, Canonica GW, Simons FE, et al. Consensus Group on New-Generation Antihistamines (CONGA): Present status and recommendations. Clin Exp Allergy. 2003;33:1305-24.
19. Yanai K, Zhang D, Tashiro M, et al. Positron emission tomography evaluation of sedative properties of antihistamines. Expert Opin Drug Saf. 2011;10:613-22.
20. Hiraoka K, Tashiro M, Grobosch T, et al. Brain histamine H1 receptor occupancy measured by PET after oral administration of levocetirizine, a non-sedating antihistamine. Expert Opin Drug Saf. 2015;14:199-206.
21. Weller K, Ziege C, Staubach P, et al. H1-antihistamine up-dosing in chronic spontaneous urticaria: Patients' perspective of effectiveness and side effects—a retrospective survey study. PLoS One. 2011;6:e23931.
22. Farre M, Perez-Mana C, Papaseit E, et al. Bilastine vs. hydroxyzine: Occupation of brain histamine H1-receptors evaluated by positron emission tomography in healthy volunteers. Br J Clin Pharmacol. 2014;78:970-80.
23. Miura M, Uno T. Clinical pharmacokinetics of fexofenadine enantiomers. Expert Opin Drug Metab Toxicol. 2010;6:69-74.
24. Church MK. Safety and efficacy of bilastine: A new H(1)-antihistamine for the treatment of allergic rhinoconjunctivitis and urticaria. Expert Opin Drug Saf. 2011;10:779-93.
25. Church MK, Labeaga L. Bilastine: A new H1-antihistamine with an optimal profile for updosing in urticaria. J Eur Acad Dermatol Venereol. 2017;31:1447-52.
26. Church MK, Kolkhir P, Metz M, et al. The role and relevance of mast cells in urticaria. Immunol Rev. 2018;282:232-47.
27. Petersen LJ, Church MK, Skov PS. Histamine is released in the wheal but not the flare following challenge of human skin in vivo: A microdialysis study. Clin Exp Allergy. 1997;27:284-95.
28. Church MK, Bewley AP, Clough GF, et al. Studies into the mechanisms of dermal inflammation using cutaneous microdialysis. Int Arch Allergy Immunol. 1997;113:131-3.
29. Maurer M, Weller K, Bindslev-Jensen C, et al. Unmet clinical needs in chronic spontaneous urticaria. A GA(2)LEN task force report. Allergy. 2011;66:317-30.
30. Zuberbier T, Aberer W, Asero R, et al. The EAACI/GA(2)LEN/EDF/WAO guideline for the definition, classification, diagnosis and management of urticaria. Allergy. 2018;73:1393-414.
31. Church MK, Maurer M. H(1)-antihistamines and urticaria: How can we predict the best drug for our patient? Clin Exp Allergy. 2012;42:1423-9.
32. Grant JA, Riethuisen JM, Moulaert B, et al. A double-blind, randomized, single-dose, crossover comparison of levocetirizine with ebastine, fexofenadine, loratadine, mizolastine, and placebo: Suppression of histamine-induced wheal-and-flare response during 24 hours in healthy male subjects. Ann Allergy Asthma Immunol. 2002;88:190-7.

33. Denham KJ, Boutsiouki P, Clough GF, et al. Comparison of the effects of desloratadine and levocetirizine on histamine-induced wheal, flare and itch in human skin. Inflamm Res. 2003;52:424-7.
34. Purohit A, Melac M, Pauli G, et al. Comparative activity of cetirizine and desloratadine on histamine-induced wheal-and-flare responses during 24 hours. Ann Allergy Asthma Immunol. 2004;92:635-40.
35. Purohit A, Melac M, Pauli G, et al. Twenty-four-hour activity and consistency of activity of levocetirizine and desloratadine in the skin. Br J Clin Pharmacol. 2003;56:388-94.
36. Purohit A, Duvernelle C, Melac M, et al. Twenty-four hours of activity of cetirizine and fexofenadine in the skin. Ann Allergy Asthma Immunol. 2001;86:387-92.
37. Lucero ML, Gonzalo A, Ganza A, et al. Interactions of bilastine, a new oral H(1) antihistamine, with human transporter systems. Drug Chem Toxicol. 2012;35:8-17.
38. Krause K, Spohr A, Zuberbier T, et al. Up-dosing with bilastine results in improved effectiveness in cold contact urticaria. Allergy. 2013;68:921-8.
39. Gray SL, Anderson ML, Dublin S, et al. Cumulative use of strong anticholinergics and incident dementia: A prospective cohort study. JAMA Intern Med. 2015;175:401-7.
40. Farré M, Bullich S, Pérez-Mañá C, et al. Brain histamine H1-receptor occupancy of bilastine, a new second-generation antihistamine, measured by positron emission tomography. Basic Clin Pharmacol Toxicol. 2013;113:12-12.

CHAPTER 8

Treatment of Chronic Spontaneous Urticaria

Kiran V Godse

INTRODUCTION

Urticaria is a heterogeneous group of diseases. All types and subtypes of urticaria share a common distinctive skin reaction pattern, i.e. the development of urticarial skin lesions and/or angioedema. Urticaria needs to be differentiated from other medical conditions where wheals can occur as a symptom, e.g. skin prick test or acute anaphylaxis without symptoms in daily life. Chronic urticaria has a spectrum of clinical presentations and causes. About 25–45% of patients have histamine-releasing autoantibodies in their blood. The term autoimmune urticaria is increasingly being accepted for this subgroup of patients. The term autoimmune urticaria is used to reflect advances in knowledge about functional autoantibodies that activate mast cells and basophils through cross linking high affinity immunoglobulin E (IgE) receptors to secrete histamine.

DEFINITION

Urticaria is characterized by the rapid appearance of wheals and/or angioedema.

A wheal consists of three typical features: (1) a central swelling of variable size, almost invariably surrounded by a reflex erythema; (2) associated itching or sometimes burning sensations; and (3) a transient nature, with the skin returning to its normal appearance, usually within 1–24 hours.

Classification of the urticarial diseases is based on duration and frequency. The timeline of 6 weeks of daily or nearly daily symptoms has been chosen as the arbitrary dividing point between acute and chronic urticaria (CU). This classification has been useful for appropriate differential diagnosis, as common causes of acute and CU are different and the two conditions behave differently.

MANAGEMENT OF CHRONIC URTICARIA

Urticaria has a profound impact on the quality of life and causes immense distress to patients, necessitating effective treatment.

The management of urticaria should consist of following two approaches, and both lines of treatment should be considered in every patient.
1. Identification of underlying cause (s) and/or eliciting trigger (s).
2. Treatment for symptomatic relief.

Especially for patients suffering from physical urticaria, treating underlying cause is the most desirable, but it is unfortunately not possible in the most of the patients. Avoidance of the triggering factor or stimulus is second best approach. This is possible for the rare patients with IgE-mediated urticaria and partly for patients suffering from physical urticaria.[1]

A step-by-step approach tailored to the individual patient should be taken for management of CU. Routine management of autoimmune and non-autoimmune CU is the same.[2]

GENERAL MEASURES

Aspirin is the most common drug to aggravate urticaria. Aspirin and other nonsteroidal anti-inflammatory drugs (NSAIDs) can worsen CU in 20–30% of patients during active phase but probably not in remission. Number of aggravating factors of urticaria can be avoided by simple measures. Treating physicians can identify these triggers or aggravating factors by taking careful history from the patient. The aggravating factors may include diet, drugs, alcohol, viral infections, local heat and friction, and mental stress.[3] In India, diet is often considered as a cause of any skin allergy. Patients often come to physician with a list of "not to eat" items. Pseudoallergens may be important cause of urticaria in some patients. Pseudoallergic reactions to additives, natural salicylates, and aromatic compounds are mostly dose related. At present we do not know how much is to be ingested to precipitate an attack. In an earlier study by Zuberbier et al. only 19% of patients reacted severely to challenge capsules containing food additives.[4] Although, there are no published studies on food items causing urticaria, in the clinical practice, it has been observed that tomato, wine, herbs, and nuts can worsen urticaria.

Overheating and local pressure because of belts and clothing may aggravate CU. Often there is an overlap between physical urticaria and CU. Urticaria may be worsened by alcohol because of the vasodilatation.

Viral infections may also aggravate urticaria. Upregulation of cytokines with the acute phase response causing temporary state of enhanced mast cell releasability may be the underlying mechanism for aggravation of urticaria during viral infections.[3] Treatment of identifiable cause, avoidance of triggers, advice and written information about the condition, and antihistamines treatment should be part of treatment plan. Soothing agents, such as calamine lotion give excellent symptomatic relief.

INFECTIONS AND URTICARIA

Chronic urticaria is frequently flared by viral infections. The incidence of bacterial infections such as dental sepsis, sinusitis, gallbladder, and urinary tract infection varies in different series.[5,6] Fungal infections such as onychomycosis, tinea pedis, and Candida have been considered as possible associations.[7] Chronic urticaria has been associated with parasitic infestations, such as strongyloidiasis, giardiasis, and amebiasis, particularly in developing and underdeveloped countries.[8]

While it is important to eliminate the infectious cause, such elimination may not always lead to remission of urticaria.

ANTIHISTAMINES

They are the first-line treatment for all patients with CU. Classic H_1-antihistamines with sedation as a side effect include chlorpheniramine, hydroxyzine, and diphenhydramine, etc. Newer H_1-antihistamines include fexofenadine, loratadine, desloratadine, cetirizine, levocetirizine, ebastine, mizolastine, olopatadine, rupatadine, etc.; H_2-antihistamines include ranitidine and famotidine. In some cases of CU, the combination of H_2-antihistamines may prove effective.

First-generation antihistamines can interfere with rapid eye movement (REM) sleep and impact on learning and performance. New GA²LEN/EDF/EAACI/WAO guidelines recommend against the use of these sedating antihistamines for the routine management of CU as the first-line agents (Fig. 8.1).[1] Thus, considering good safety profile of second generation antihistamines they should be considered as the first-line symptomatic treatment for urticaria. Higher dosing of second-generation antihistamines have been shown to be effective in control of chronic spontaneous urticaria. This has been verified in studies using even up to four-fold higher than recommended doses of desloratadine,[9] fexofenadine,[10] levocetirizine,[11] and rupatadine.[12]

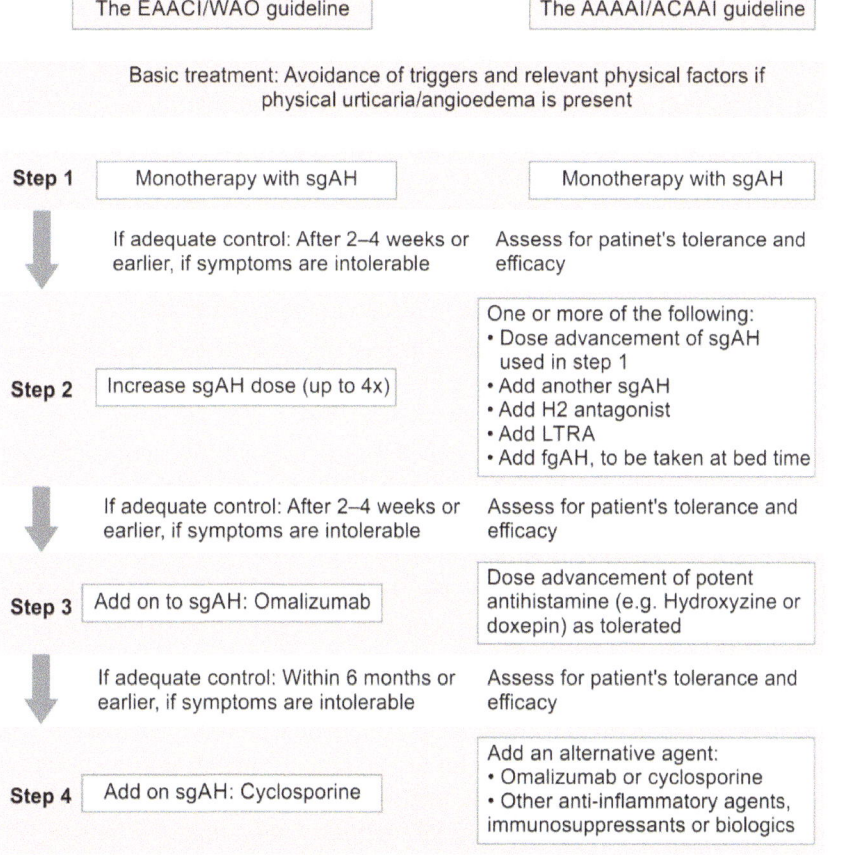

Fig. 8.1: Comparison of EAACI/WAO/GA2LEN/EDF guidelines with American guidelines.
(EAACI: European Academy of Allergy and Clinical Immunology; WAO: World Allergy Organization; AAAAI: American Academy of Allergy, Asthma & Immunology; ACAAI: American College of Allergy, Asthma, and Immunology)

While antihistamines up to four times the manufacturers' recommended dosages will control symptoms in the majority of patients with urticaria in general practice, alternative treatments are needed for the remaining unresponsive patients.

Hydroxyzine is efficacious in relieving pruritus in various forms of eczema and dermatitis and urticaria. Hydroxyzine is derivative of piperazine not related to phenothiazines. Hydroxyzine is more effective than nsAHs when given as recommended dose in suppressing histamine-induced wheal or allergic skin reactions.[13] Hydroxyzine reduces anxiety by suppression of activity in certain key regions of the subcortical area of the CNS. This drug is useful in anxiety associated with urticaria. Journal of Allergy and Clinical Immunology (JACI) guidelines mentions addition of sedating antihistamine to be taken at bedtime as step 2 in guidelines.

Montelukast (leukotriene antagonist) is useful in aspirin-induced urticaria or in patients with positive autologous serum skin test. Those patients who have associated respiratory allergies such as allergic rhinitis or asthma benefit from montelukast therapy.

H_2-antihistamines can be added along with H_1-antihistamines for synergistic effect. There are no randomized controlled trials available of this combination.

Dapsone is an antibacterial sulfonamide with anti-inflammatory properties. This drug is effective in delayed pressure urticaria. Dapsone is available as 100 mg tablet to be taken once a day. Before starting dapsone therapy complete blood count and G6PD test should be done.

Doxepin is a tricyclic antidepressant with strong antihistaminic effect. Doxepin is effective if sleep is disturbed due to itching. JACI guidelines published in 2014 mentions hydroxyzine and doxepin as step 3 approach in CU.

At present, corticosteroids are frequently used in allergic diseases. There is a strong recommendation from GA²LEN/EDF/EAACI/WAO guidelines against the long-term use of corticosteroids outside specialist clinics if it can be avoided.[1] A dose of 0.5 mg/kg/day of prednisolone can be used for up to 1 week to resolve acute exacerbation.

Cyclosporine has a moderate, direct effect on mast cell mediator release.[14] It is recommended only for patients with severe disease refractory to maximum dose of antihistamines. Cyclosporine has a far better risk/benefit ratio compared with steroids.

Cyclosporine has been reported to be beneficial in many studies; some of the studies were double blind controlled studies. In some studies, the dose of cyclosporine used was between 4 mg and 5 mg/kg, whereas a low dose (2–3 mg/kg) was given in the other studies.[15] Generally, cyclosporine is given for up to 3 months.

Methotrexate may be a useful and cost-effective alternative for steroid-dependent CU in the Indian settings.[16] Functional autoantibodies do not correlate with the response to treatment. The beneficial effects of methotrexate are due to its anti-inflammatory and immunosuppressive properties. Methotrexate can be used up to 10–15 mg/week for its steroids sparing effect.[17]

Omalizumab is a recombinant, humanized, monoclonal antibody against IgE. Omalizumab acts as a neutralizing antibody by binding IgE at the same site on IgE as its high-affinity receptor (FcRI). Omalizumab reduces serum levels of IgE and blocks the attachment of IgE to mast cells and other immune cells, thereby preventing IgE-mediated inflammatory changes. Omalizumab is approved for the treatment of moderate-to-severe persistent asthma in adults and adolescents older than 12 years of age who have a positive skin test to a perennial allergen. Dosing is based on weight and pretreatment serum IgE levels and is administered via subcutaneous injection every 2–4 weeks. Injection site reaction is the most commonly reported adverse event with omalizumab. Omalizumab (anti-IgE) has now been shown to be dramatically effective in selected patients with chronic spontaneous urticaria.[18] Omalizumab is now approved by US FDA, EMA, and DGCI of India for use in CU.

Now we know response to omalizumab can be divided in two groups.
1. *Subgroup one*: Early treatment responders—patients who responded after one dose of omalizumab (<4 weeks).
2. *Subgroup two*: Late treatment responders—patients who need additional time to respond (up to 24 weeks).

Increased IgE levels linked to faster relapse in omalizumab discontinued CU patients.
- Omalizumab
- Prevents angioedema development
- Markedly improves quality of life
- It is suitable for long-term treatment
- It effectively treats relapse after discontinuation omalizumab, in CU, is effective at doses from 150–300 mg/month.

Patients seem to have a higher probability to respond to omalizumab if they have high baseline serum IgE levels, low D-dimer levels and no intake of ACE inhibitors. Patients with autologous serum skin test positive takes longer time to respond to omalizumab.

Autologous serum therapy has been found to be successful in CU in an Indian study.[19] Larger studies are required to confirm findings. Autohemotherapy can induce tolerization/desensitization of autoreactive CU patients to the proinflammatory signals expressed in their circulation.

A strong recommendation was made by the GA²LEN/EDF/EAACI/WAO panel to discourage the use of first-generation antihistamines in infants and children. Thus, in children, the same first-line treatment and updosing (weight adjusted) is recommended as in adults.[1]

In pregnancy, we suggest the use of second-generation antihistamines should be limited to loratadine and levocetirizine. The increased dosage of second-generation antihistamines can only be carefully suggested in pregnancy since safety studies have not been done. While using loratadine, it must be remembered that it is metabolized in the liver. First-generation agents may be used cautiously when symptoms are nonresponsive to second-generation antihistamines during pregnancy.

According to the data from Berlin Teratogen Information Service, 196 women exposed in any trimester (11% in the first trimester), showed no increased risk of birth defects or other adverse outcomes with cetirizine. Maternal use of loratadine, desloratadine, or fexofenadine in a standard therapeutic dose is unlikely to result in adverse effects in nursing infants due to minimal exposure of a nursing infant to the drugs through breast milk.[20]

Safety of second-generation antihistamines should be considered when these drugs are to be used in patients with liver disease, renal impairment and in geriatric patients. Table 8.1 lists the metabolism and dose adjustment of various second-generation antihistamines.[14,21]

Controversial areas between US and international guidelines are:
- Pseudoallergen-free diet
- First-generation sedating antihistamines.

The international guidelines (GA²LEN/EDF/EAACI/WAO) strongly advise against the use of first-generation sedating antihistamines on the basis of high level of evidence for adverse

Table 8.1: Metabolism and dose adjustment of various second generation antihistamines.

Drug	Liver metabolism	Dose adjustment
Fexofenadine	<8%	Kidney failure
Levocetirizine	<15%	Liver and kidney failure
Desloratadine	Yes	Liver and kidney failure
Rupatadine	Yes	Liver and kidney failure
Cetirizine	<40%	Liver and kidney failure
Loratadine	Yes	Liver and kidney failure

Flowchart 8.1: Indian consensus statement on urticaria.

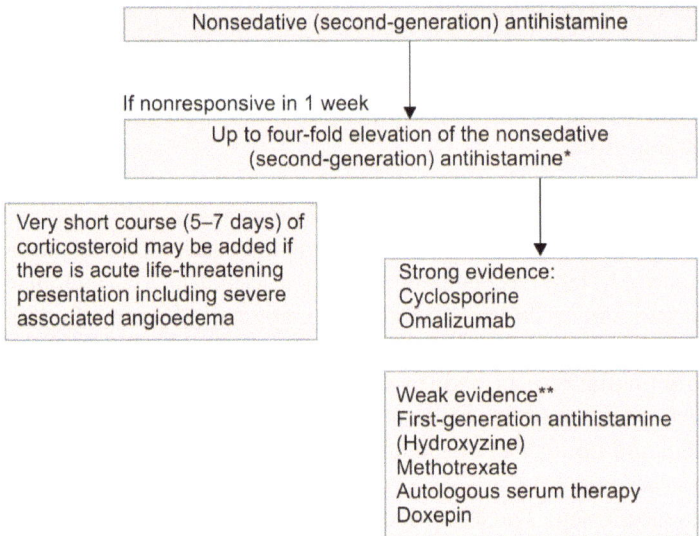

*Safety evidence of up-dosing is available for levocetirizine, desloratadine and fexofenadine
**May be considered in selected situation.

events and no studies demonstrating greater efficacy than second-generation antihistamines (*see* Fig. 8.1).[22,23]

This is Indian consensus statement for urticarial management published in 2018 (Flowchart 8.1).[24]

REFERENCES

1. Zuberbier T, Aberer W, Asero R, et al. EAACI/GA2LEN/ EDF/WAO Guideline for the definition, classification, diagnosis, and management of urticaria: the 2013 revision and update. Allergy. 2014;69:868-87.
2. Yadav S, Upadhyay A, Bajaj AK. Chronic urticaria: An overview. Indian J Dermatol. 2006;51:171-7.
3. Grattan C. Chronic urticaria: General principles and management. In: Greaves MW, Kaplan AP (Eds). Urticaria and Angioedema. New York: Marcel Dekker; 2009. pp.346-9.
4. Zuberbier T, Chantraine-Hess S, Hartmann K, et al. Pseudoallergen free diet in the treatment of chronic urticaria. Acta Derm Venereol. 1995;75:484-7.

5. Pasricha JS, Kanwar AJ. Survey of the causes of urticaria. Indian J Dermatol Venereol Leprol. 1979;45:6-12.
6. Kaur S, Ghosh S, Kanwar AJ, et al. Incidence of dental caries in chronic urticaria. Indian J Dermatol Venereol Leprol. 1991;57:276-8.
7. James J, Warin RP. An assessment of the role of *Candida albicans* and food yeast in chronic urticaria. Br J Dermatol. 1971;84:227-37.
8. Ghosh S, Kanwar AJ, Dhar S, et al. Role of gastrointestinal parasites in urticaria. Indian J Dermatol Venereol Leprol. 1993;59:117-9.
9. Siebenhaar F, Degener F, Zuberbier T, et al High-dose desloratadine decreases wheat volume and improves cold provocation thresholds as compared with standard dose treatment in patients with acquired cold urticaria: a randomized, placebo-controlled, crossover study. J Allergy Clin Immunol. 2009;123:672-9.
10. Godse KV, Nadkarni NJ, Jani G, et al. Fexofenadine in higher doses in chronic spontaneous urticaria. Indian Dermatol Online J. 2010;1:45-6.
11. Godse KV. Updosing of antihistamines to improve control of chronic urticaria. Indian J Dermatol Venereol Leprol. 2010;76:61-2.
12. Godse K. Allergic diseases of the skin and drug allergies—2022. Consensus statement on management of urticaria in India. World Allergy Organ J. 2013;6:109-10.
13. Gimenez-Arnau A, Izquierdo I, Maurer M. The use of a responder analysis to identify clinically meaningful differences in chronic urticaria patients following placebo-controlled treatment with rupatadine 10 and 20 mg. J Eur Acad Dermatol Venereol. 2009;23:1088-91.
14. So M, Bozzo P, Inoue M, et al. Safety of antihistamines during pregnancy and lactation. Can Fam Physician. 2010;56:427-9.
15. dos Santos RV, Magerl M, Mlynek A, et al. Suppression of histamine- and allergen-induced skin reactions: comparison of first- and second-generation antihistamines. Ann Allergy Asthma Immunol. 2009;102:495-9.
16. Kessel A, Toubi E. Cyclosporine-A in severe chronic urticaria: the option for long-term therapy. Allergy. 2010;65:1478-82.
17. Godse K. Methotrexate in autoimmune urticaria. Indian J Dermatol Venereol Leprol. 2004;70:377.
18. Perez A, Woods A, Grattan CE, et al. Methotrexate: A useful steroid-sparing agent in recalcitrant chronic urticaria. Br J Dermatol. 2010;162:191-4.
19. Godse KV. Omalizumab in severe chronic urticaria. Indian J Dermatol Venereol Leprol. 2008;74:157-8.
20. Bajaj AK, Saraswat A, Upadhyay A, et al. Autologous serum therapy in chronic urticaria: Old wine in a new bottle. Indian J Dermatol Venereol Leprol. 2008;74:109-13.
21. del Cuvillo A, Mullol J, Bartra J, et al. Comparative pharmacology of the H1 antihistamines. J Investig Allergol Clin Immunol. 2006;16:3-12.
22. Bernstein JA, Lang DM, Khan DA, et al. The diagnosis and management of acute and chronic urticaria: 2014 update. J Allergy Clin Immunol. 2014;133:1270-7.
23. Zuberbier T, Bernstein JA. A comparison of the United States and international perspective on chronic urticaria guidelines. J Allergy Clin Immunol Pract. 2018;6:1144-51.
24. Godse K, De A, Zawar V, et al. Consensus statement for the diagnosis and treatment of urticaria: A 2017 update. Indian J Dermatol. 2018;63:2-15

Annexure

UAS7* is a weekly composite score of the ISS and number of hives score, used to measure disease activity[1]
- Weekly ISS is the sum of daily ISS over 7 days (scale 0–21)
- Weekly number of hives score is the sum of the daily number of hives score over 7 days (scale 0–21)
- UAS7 is a composite score of the weekly ISS and weekly number of hives score (scale 0–42)

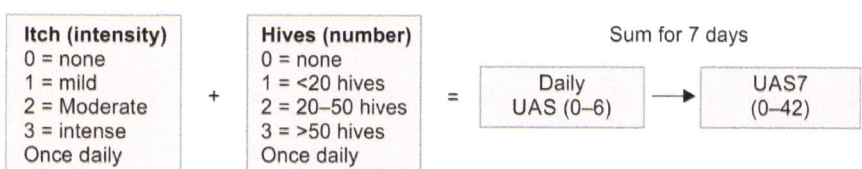

*AS recommended in the 2013 urticaria CAACI/GA^{2}LEN/EDF/WAO guidelines
1. Adapted from: Zuberbier T, et al. Allergy. 2014;69:868-87.
(ISS: Itch Severity Score; UAS: Urticaria Activity Score; UAS7: Weekly Urticaria Activity Score)

URTICARIA CONTROL TEST (UCT)

Instruction: You are suffering from nettle rash (urticaria). The following questions will record your current disease activity. Please read each question carefully and from the five answers select the one that best applies for you. Please refer to the last 4 weeks. Do not think about it for long and remember to answer all questions and select only one answer for each question.

1. How much have you suffered from the physical symptoms of urticaria (itching, wheals and/or swelling) in the last 4 weeks?
   Very severely   severely   moderately   a little   not at all

2. How greatly did the urticaria interfere with your quality of life in the last 4 weeks?
   Very severely   severely   moderately   a little   not at all

3. How often in the last 4 weeks was the treatment for your urticaria insufficient to control the urticaria symptoms?
   Very often   often   occasionally   rarely   not at all

4. How well did you have your urticaria under control overall in the last 4 weeks?
   Not at all   hardly at all   moderately   well   completely

The urticaria is regarded as controlled with a UCT of > 12 points and as uncontrolled ≤ 11 points.
©MOXIE GmbH, www.moxie-gmbh.de

URTICARIA CAN BE CLASSIFIED BASED ON DURATION, FREQUENCY, AND CAUSE[1]

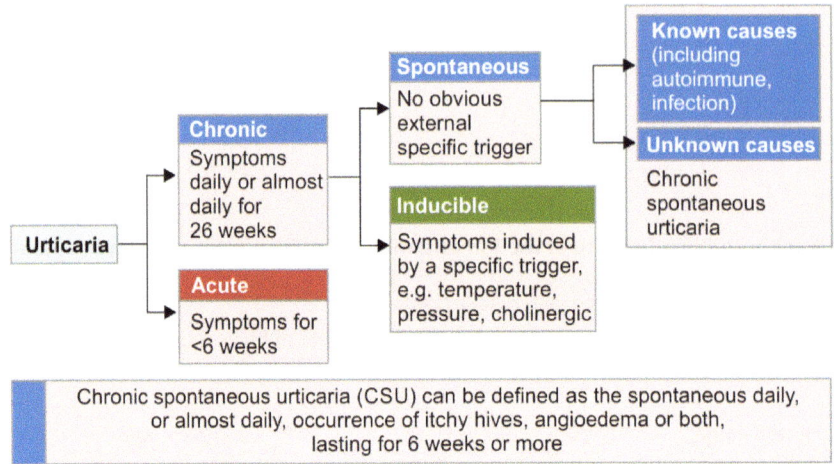

1. Adapted from: Zuberbier T, et al. Allergy. 2014;69:868-87.

Index

Page numbers followed by f refer to figure, and t refer to table

A

Acetylcholine, effects of 62
Acetylsalicylic acid 40
American Academy of Allergy, Asthma & Immunology 71
American College of Allergy, Asthma, and Immunology 71
Angioedema 1-3, 5, 44, 45, 47f, 49
  acquired 2, 3, 48, 49
  cell-dependent 45
  classification 45
  differential diagnosis of 49
  epidemiology 45
  etiology of 46
  hereditary 1-3, 44, 46, 49
  management 50
  mast cell-independent 50
  non-histaminergic 3
  pathogenesis 45
  spontaneous 48
Angiotensin converting enzyme 2
  inhibitors 49
Antibodies, antinuclear 8
Antihistamines 71
  action of 65
  first-generation 71
  pharmacology of 62
Antistreptolysin test 8
Aspirin 70
Autoinflammatory disease 2
Autologous serum skin test 6, 6f

B

Bilastine 66
Blood-brain barrier 63

C

Cardiovascular symptoms 59
Central nervous system 63
Cetirizine 66, 71, 74
C-reactive protein 8
Cutaneous mastocytosis 3, 54, 55, 60
  classification 54
  clinical features 55
  complications 59
  course 60
  diagnosis 57
  differential diagnosis 58
  epidemiology 55
  etiology 55
  investigations 57
  pathogenesis 55
  prognosis 60
  treatment 59
Cyclosporins 72

D

Dapsone 72
Darier's sign 56, 56f
Dementia 66
Dermographism, asymptomatic 3t, 10, 14, 32, 33f
Desloratadine 71, 74
Diarrhea 59

E

Ebastine 71
Eczema 23, 24f
Erythrocyte sedimentation rate 8, 49
European Academy of Allergy and Clinical Immunology 71

F

Fexofenadine 66, 71, 74
Fibrin degradation products 47

G

Giemsa stain 58f

H

Helicobacter pylori 9, 52
Heterogeneous disease 54
Histamine 63
    antagonists 62
Histaminergic transmission 63

I

Immunoglobulin E 8, 46
Itchy wheals 5

K

Kinin-mediated angioedema, treatment of 51t

L

Leukotriene antagonist 72
Levocetirizine 66, 71, 74
Loratadine 71, 74

M

Mast cell 57
    activating antibodies 8
    dependent angioedema 45, 50
    derived histamine 64
    independent angioedema 46
Mastocytoma, solitary 56f
Mastocytosis 57f
    classification of 54f
    systemic 58
Metachromatic granules 58f
Methotrexate 72
Mimicking xanthoma 59f
Mizolastine 71
Molecular weight
    high 20, 47
    low 20
Mucous membranes 1

N

Nausea 59
Nettle rash 78
Nonsteroidal anti-inflammatory drugs 7, 40, 46, 70

O

Olopatadine 71
Omalizumab 72

P

Plasma concentration 65
Polymorphic pigmented lesions 56f
Protein contact dermatitis 20
Pseudoallergic reactions 7

R

Rapid eye movement 71
Reticulate erythema 44
Rupatadine 71, 74

S

Shock 59
Skin
    lesions, sudden urtication of 56
    mast cells 57
    prick test 24, 69
    provocation tests 7
Solar urticaria 10, 14, 16, 28-31, 35f
Sporadic disorder 55
Steroids, anabolic 53
Syncope 59

T

Telangiectasia macularis eruptiva perstans 57
TempTest® device, use of 13f
Tranexamic acid 50, 53

U

Urtica obonica 21
Urticaria 1, 3, 5, 12f, 64, 69, 70, 79
    activity score 9t
    acute spontaneous 5
    allergic 2

aquagenic 17, 28, 29, 31, 32, 40
   clinical features 40
   diagnosis 40
   epidemiology 40
   treatment 40
causal 79
cholinergic 2, 11f, 14, 16, 17, 28, 29, 31, 32, 38
   clinical features 39
   diagnosis 39
   epidemiology 39
   treatment 39
chronic 65, 69, 70
   inducible 28, 28t-31t
   spontaneous 3, 5, 7, 8, 9t, 28, 64, 69
classification of 1, 2
cold 10, 13, 28, 30, 31, 33
   clinical features 34
   diagnosis 34
   epidemiology 33
   treatment 35
contact 2, 10, 17, 20
   diagnosis 22
   physiopathology 21
   treatment for 25
control test 78
delayed pressure 10, 14, 28-31, 36
   clinical features 37
   diagnosis 37
   epidemiology 37
   treatment 37
diagnosis of 5
duration 79
factitia 10, 14, 16f, 32
familial cold 3
form of 12, 14
frequency 79
heat 10, 28, 29, 30, 31, 36
   clinical features 36
   diagnosis 36
   epidemiology 36
   treatment 36
inducible 10
management of 70
manifestation of 1
physical 70
pigmentosa 3, 55, 55f, 59
pressure 3, 15f
severe cold 34f
solar 37
   clinical features 37
   diagnosis 38
   epidemiology 37
   treatment 38
spontaneous 50
subtypes of 3
symptom of 1
syndrome 20
   contact 20, 22, 25
types of 64
vasculitis 3
vibratory 10, 17
Urticarial diseases, classification of 69

V

Vibratory angioedema 17, 28, 29, 31, 39
   clinical features 38
   diagnosis 38
   epidemiology 38
   treatment 38
Viral infections 70
Vomiting 59

W

World Allergy Organization 71

Printed by Libri Plureos GmbH in Hamburg, Germany